CW01034386

THE BODY PLAN

SIMPLE, EFFECTIVE AND FLEXIBLE STRATEGIES
FOR PERMANENT WEIGHT LOSS IN THE
REAL WORLD

ROBYN LAW

RPMC

FREE BONUS RECIPE BOOK INVITATION

Sign up to receive a free ebook of my favourite recipes and a meal plan to get you started and complement the strategies I share in *The Body Plan*.

http://bit.ly/bodyplanrecipes

For Patrick, Manus and Chloé

WHAT OTHERS ARE SAYING

"Thanks so much for your inspiration and for showing me how I can lose weight without cutting out all the "bad" stuff! As a busy working mum, I don't have much time for exercise. I lost almost 20kg just by changing my diet alone and learning about portion control. Thanks Robyn!"

Kylie Wood, Cairns, Queensland

"Thank you, Robyn, for putting yourself out there and being so honest and so 'real'. You have inspired me to step out of my comfort zone and reach for a better version of myself."

Teila Jarlowe, United States & Saudi Arabia

"Having never dieted in my life, I was very sceptical as to whether I could actually stick to Robyn's plan. Seeing Robyn's transformation is enough to get anyone to 'believe'. It took me a while to get the hang of the whole tracking my food criteria, but after three weeks I figured it out and got the hang of it. Her game plan really gets you thinking about what you eat and how every spoon, bite, the choice makes a difference. If you want that slice of cake, eat it, but then don't expect to be able to eat a carb-filled meal at dinner time. It's all about balance and compromise. I didn't need to lose a drastic amount of weight. I achieved the little that I needed. But what I did gain was knowledge, confidence in myself that I could be persistent during the whole program and I learnt about balance. Thanks, Robyn for the valuable support, training and opening my eyes to how we really should look at food."

Mara Mostafa, United Arab Emirates & Bahrain

"Robyn's book has transformed weight loss into a manageable and easy to follow solution that gets results. I love that her plan follows a realistic path to genuine results - unlike previous plans I've followed which required serious deprivation. I would definitely recommend her book to anyone who has struggled in the past to stick to a program - this book will change your way of thinking about your health and give you practical tools to implement for lasting change!"

Megan Taz, Brisbane, Australia

"Robyn taught me to be kind to myself while still loving my body and my body journey. She gave me the tools to lose weight while still enjoying the foods I love. She is supportive and motivational as needed. Can't wait to read this book & continue my journey!"

Jessica, Sydney, Australia

I would like to thank you! For your words of wisdom and encouragement that I seem to need quite often when I was ready to give up. You are truly a role model for your children, family and friends.

Rommleigh, Saudi Arabia

ABOUT THE AUTHOR

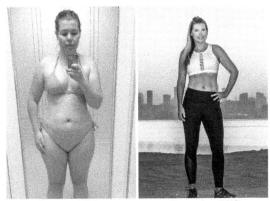

January 2016   December 2017

Robyn Law is an Australian expat living with her husband and two children in the Middle East.

In 2002, Robyn was inspired to give up her safe and reliable corporate career in finance to take a year off city life and get paid to travel as a 'glamorous' flight attendant with Richard Branson's newly formed Australian branch of *Virgin Airlines*.

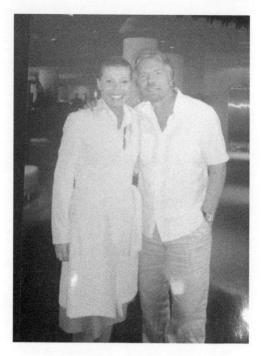

Robyn and Richard Branson, 2005

Three years later, still flying and loving it, Robyn embarked on a world adventure after bearing witness to friends settling down and starting families with nothing resembling this looming on her horizon.

After a varied professional life including nannying, stints in television and corporate management roles, she found herself back where she really thrived, in the skies for Australian airline *QANTAS*, based out of London, flying to South East Asia every week.

Being paid to party and sleep was fun, but when she was offered a top-tier role working on a private jet shortly after hitting the big thirty, she jumped at the chance, to bank tax-free cash and have an enforced 'detox' in dry and restricted Saudi Arabia.

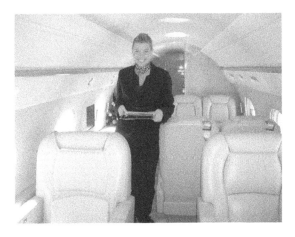

Saudi Arabia, 2008

Living and working in Saudi Arabia, flying diplomats and oil company management all over the world was a once in a lifetime opportunity, but the real payoff was the paid downtime which was when Robyn first discovered the new world of blogging; documenting her worldwide travels and adventures.

Her blogging organically morphed into a popular and professional health and wellness site, *Girl on Raw,* resulting in Robyn travelling to the US to officially train as a *Raw Food Chef,* being named by *Australian Woman's Day* magazine as *Australia's Leading Raw Chef* in 2014.

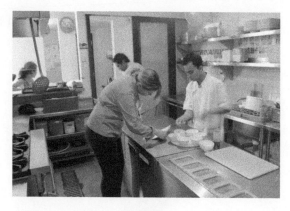

Bali, 2014

No longer a practising raw foodie, but evolving as a continual student of self-transformation, health, nutrition, fitness, and self-development through formal training and self-study, Robyn hopes to inspire through sharing her own unique journey, mistakes and lessons acquired from her varied careers, international travel and exposure to a wide variety of cultures and people.

Plus, she just loves to write, eat, cook, train, travel and live her best life!

Disclaimer
The information in this book is based on the author's personal journey, research, lifestyle and experience. She is sharing this for educational, informational and sometimes entertainment purposes only. Please conduct your own research and consult your own doctor or healthcare provider to determine the best course of action for you.

instagram.com/robynjlaw

amazon.com/author/robynlaw

CONTENTS

FOREWORD

Transformation can occur in more than one way. We can transform how we look, how we behave, how we think about the world, and even genetically alter our cells – the inner workings of the body.

For as long as I've known Robyn, she's been transforming. From her education to her professional careers, to her wardrobe, she's always evolving – and the beauty of evolution is that it never ends. There's still something new to learn, to do, to be; and this is part of the excitement of transformation.

When Robyn first embarked on this journey, I knew it wasn't going to be a small one. I knew it was going to be a big, life-changing journey that would transform every aspect of her life. Most importantly, as a friend, the transformation I most wished for, was for her to find peace and self-love.

Watching your best friend feel uncomfortable in front of the camera, and be in constant nagging back pain, and be unhappy in so many areas of her life isn't easy. No amount of, 'You look amazing!' or 'You don't need to lose weight!' helps when the problem is deeper than that. And the problem did run deeper.

When she told me she was heading offline for a break (and

isn't it ironic that we often 'surf the net' for a break from our day-to-day, where now we seek respite from the onslaught of the online world?!), I knew she was serious. She needed to go deep. She needed to go within. No more comparing the lives, bodies, looks, or wealth of unknown strangers online. No more falling down the rabbit hole and gasping to come up for air.

This was it. This was the beginning. This was when I knew Robyn was doing it for herself.

It wasn't for validation or approval from anyone. It was all for herself. And there's power in that; so much more power than when you're seeking something for a superficial reason.

I watched and waited. I held space for Robyn, from across the seas. I knew it was happening – on a soul level, I could feel her shift, her evolution and her spark coming back.

I've always told Robyn how beautiful she is. I often tried to bolster her – in my eyes, she didn't need to change. She was still beautiful. But her happiness and health were necessary to come first. So, I shelved my opinion that she didn't need to change and helped her embrace it instead.

The transformation was well underway, and I began to notice more than just a slimming down of her face during our *Skype* chats. I saw the sparkle in her eyes return. I saw confidence that had been hidden under layers of everyday life re-emerge. I heard her voice, the strength and power clearly stating what she wanted.

Her children had a happy mum. Her husband had a happy wife. I had a happy friend! And it was the heartfelt kind of happiness that comes from true self-love and worth.

Most importantly, she had peace. A calmness was surrounding her that hadn't been there before. It seemed to emanate from her and wash over everything like calming waves. It was a relief. To see peace in what before were rough seas was magical.

And I know that her magic will help you transform your life as well.

Adele McConnell

Author, Creator of <u>www.vegiehead.com</u>, and vegan skincare range Dusk by Adele. Owner of organic, plant-based cafe, SoulPod Foods in Melbourne, Australia.

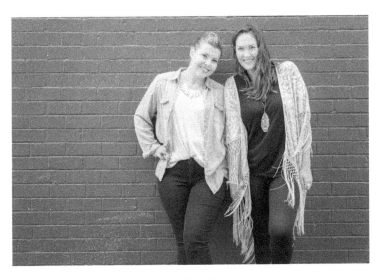

Robyn and Adele, Brisbane, 2015

MY STORY

After years experimenting with some of the most popular fad diets including juice fasts, *Atkins*, *Weight Watchers*, even accidentally creating a business around raw food education, I'm finally in a place where I have found a comfortable and sustainable balanced lifestyle centred around sensible eating.

The approach that I share in this book works perfectly for me, at this stage of life as the primary caregiver and at home mother to my two, active, growing kids and a busy, hard-working husband.

In my past, most if not all of the diets I tried required restriction. Fortunately, however, I never reached the point of an official eating disorder, although I can appreciate how some can.

Most of these somehow restrictive diets often deliver short-term success and weight loss, however, when returning to a typical way of eating, the results experienced often are reversed.

To be fair, I've never really had an extreme weight problem; however, like a lot of women, I owned a 'skinny' and 'fat' section in my wardrobe of clothes, which included two to four various dress sizes. My daily garment size would change according to my mood or season. At my heaviest, according to the *Body Mass*

(BMI) I was considered clinically obese. *BMI* standards are an estimated guide that doesn't take into account many factors; I talk more about this further in the book.

Following the birth of my second child, despite having a very healthy pregnancy I began to gain weight months after giving birth, when many other new mothers are motivated and some even effortlessly successful in dropping the baby weight.

Weight loss and body image were not on my radar as a new mother, for obvious and practical reasons. Over those years following my youngest's arrival until she was three and a half, I didn't have the mental bandwidth to focus on my own self-care, and so my weight continued to increase.

I was in denial of my weight gain, as I stepped through my daily to-do's of caring for my family, and running a part-time online business, often falling exhausted into bed at the end of the day, ready to do it all again the following day.

Until several severe events in a short space of time occurred including:

Event One: During a conversation with a good friend who is both diabetic and a diabetes nurse and educator, we discussed my strong family history of diabetes 1 and 2. My mother had recently been diagnosed at fifty-seven. We spoke of my concern of my own risk of diabetes due to its prevalence on my mother's side of the family. I wondered if it was time for me to be tested.

My friend believed it wasn't necessary. She could already tell by looking at me and my belly fat that I was pre-diabetic.

Event Two: With ongoing lower back pain and hip discomfort, most notably since having carried and delivered my two children, I had frequent visits to my chiropractor. They helped to ease the problem, but only temporarily. My chiropractor said he was happy to keep taking my money to adjust me and treat my symptoms, but recommended if I was seeking a long-term solution, I could work on fixing the cause by strengthening my core and back with something like a regular Pilates practice.

As a side note, he also made a comment about how he was surprised how strong my body and muscles felt beneath what felt like my body fat. He believed with commitment to a healthy diet and exercise, I could return to a lean and powerful body; he could already feel it beneath my flab. He basically told me to get serious and stop eating crap.

Amongst a couple of severe other family traumas, I was fast approaching forty. The grey hairs began to appear, changes to my menstrual cycle denoting 'the change' was around the corner and some extra wrinkles here and there. There was no better time to learn self-acceptance and commitment.

Acceptance of what I couldn't change in my life, and commitment to developing and improving what I could, on a daily basis, no matter how small the actions I would take towards my more significant goal.

Don't give up on you.

If we're lucky, we still have so many more years to live high-quality, impactful life with our family and friends, but it does require dedication and practice. Carving out a little quality time in your day and life now will add up to extra time and good health down the track. Wouldn't you rather be one of those old ladies playing energetically with your grandkids in the garden, or extending your time out of the nursing home?

We may not be able to stop the grey hairs or the laugh lines, but we can manipulate other factors that help us to slow down the ageing process so that we can live happier for longer with more energy and zest for life!

Let's do this!

At the time of writing this book, I have lost 20kg/44lb through sensible eating and exercise. Although 20kg is not the final weight loss goal I set out to achieve, with this weight loss success I have attracted a new quality of life and new habits that make it easier to reach my ultimate goal.

WHAT TO EXPECT FROM THIS BOOK

Chances are you are reading this book because you've been motivated into action by witnessing my very own transformation and wanted in on the secret.

I understand, because before my own journey and also during it, I found the real-life examples of women my age and stage in life were few and far between. Let's face it, there are enough twenty-somethings and often child-free inspiring women on the internet to last several lifetimes.

I desired to be motivated by mature, authentic examples of other women, both where I currently stood and where I wanted to be.

Maybe you're ready also to make some healthy lifestyle changes to improve your chances of longevity and a higher quality of life going into older age.

Believe it or not, that was and continues to be my first priority, not the leaner body, but hey that's not a bad goal to have either.

It's not a crime to desire to feel sexy, hot and vibrant no matter what age you are.

There are many teachers and coaches out there that will

help you to get the healthy and lean fit body that you desire, but if you're not ready to make the change, then when will you be?

I am not a nutritionist, nor am I am a personal trainer, but I have already lost over twenty kilograms without losing my mind or having to give up my favourite foods.

I am going to share with you in this book the principles I researched and the methods I applied to achieve sustainable weight loss without wanting to kill anyone in the process, especially my kids and husband.

I am my own guinea pig in this story, and I share with you what I learnt, curating some of the best research I could find, and how I've applied it in my own unique way.

During my transformation, I documented my entire journey into three-month phases because naturally, this is precisely the way it happened. Organically, three-monthly blocks were just the right amount of time for me to laser in on one or several focal points and master them before I would naturally move onto the next.

Let's imagine we're enjoying a coffee, tea or smoothie and I'm about to share with you the exact steps I took in the first and most crucial three-month phase of my weight loss journey. Have you got some time?

I don't believe in making change complicated or overwhelming, so having fewer objectives to focus on during each three-month phase ensured I was able to give each goal the attention and dedication it really deserved. All while increasing my knowledge and skills in that zone.

This book details the exact game plan I followed for the first three months and sets the tone for the entire transformational journey I embarked on.

"*Do less and do it best*", has been my motto throughout my journey.

I followed these basics principles and methods enclosed within and didn't succumb to the latest fad on the market. They'll always come and go. But the basics still remain the same.

HOW TO USE THIS BOOK

In this book, I outline precisely the steps I took to prepare myself for my whole-body transformation, in the lead up to the start date and the first three-month phase.

Naturally, throughout the first year of my transformation, there were adjustments and refinements, because nothing in life is static right?

To avoid unnecessarily overwhelming you by recommending you make all the lifestyle modifications immediately, I am going to share with you exactly what I did and how I did it incrementally, over time, for life-long lasting results.

I wanted to guarantee these adjustments to my lifestyle became habits; natural and automatic. Just like brushing my teeth twice a day, by gradually making these changes I knew I'd be less resistant to my lifestyle adjustments.

Over time, I naturally observed that my transformation's progress took on three-monthly cycles or phases. For example, the first three months were focused on introducing new eating and nutrition habits and theories. Once that was mastered, then the next three-month phase focused on fitness and movement, generally speaking. Months seven and beyond concentrated on refining and tweaking, almost a sense of going pro, getting leaner and stronger and deeper with nutritional knowledge for best performance.

By having a clear theme for each three-month phase, I was able to entirely focus on that theme, master it until it became second nature with little to no resistance, then build on it. This ensured long-lasting success and a lack of boredom moving forward.

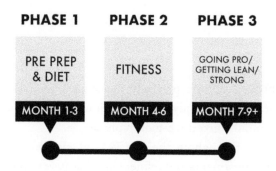

In this book, I'll be focusing on your pre-prep and months one to three.

These timelines are estimates only and may take you longer or shorter depending on your level of commitment, time available or current mindset. Please be kind to yourself and know that this is a process, there are always going to be ups and downs along the way, but it's your consistency over time that will win out in the end. As Bruce Lee said, *"Long-term consistency trumps short-term intensity."*

I think it's critical to note however that it's possible that you may not get past the first month before giving up. This resistance is to be expected for some, but don't lose heart. If that happens, depending on your desire and motivation for change, it's likely you will shortly reappear and give it another, more determined attempt.

Initially, when I came across this concept of how to transform my body, I too had a false start.

I gave up before I'd even began because the methods I share in this book, at first, seemed complicated and time-consuming. But as you'll discover in the pages ahead, just like anything worth earning it's worth sticking out. If you want to get good at something you need to keep practising.

I liken it to learning a new language or taking up a new sport or hobby. We all have to start from the beginning, but with practice and determination, you will be closer to your goal each step of the way.

This way of life is so simple and flexible for me now, full of freedom and empowerment that I would not have experienced had I not got over myself and given this an excellent shot.

Not being the expert at something immediately shouldn't derail you. Give it time, and you will become the expert of your own *body, mind* and *soul;* you just need to carve out the time to honour it.

The sooner you start, the sooner your results will show up. Don't give up before the miracle happens. A year from now, you'd have wished you started today.

To make it easier for you, I have broken this book down into three main parts.

- *My Philosophy*
- *Foundational Knowledge: Pre-prep Stage*
- *Let's Get Started: First Three Months*

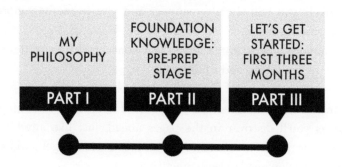

But before we begin on *My Philosophy*, you'll need to first ensure you have all the correct equipment.

Before You Get Started: Equipment Required

You can download your own checklist here in your free starter kit http://bit.ly/bodyplanstarter

Look online, visit your local stores or maybe you already have these items in your home, but these are the exact items of equipment and smartphone apps I use. Don't forget, second hand, either via thrift shops or online marketplaces is a very environmental and often an economical and responsible way to shop too. Perhaps even a family member might have some of these, unused and lying around.

You'll need these items before getting started. Make sure to allow adequate time to acquire these items before you set your kick-off date, including a week or so beforehand to allow time to record your current eating habits as outlined in *Chapter 3: Keeping Records.*

1. Journal or notebook

To register your notes and weekly check-in results. If you

prefer you can use an online spreadsheet or download a copy of my own template in your free starter kit. I personally prefer to keep manual records as well as a file on my computer.

You can download your own check-in spreadsheet here in your free starter kit http://bit.ly/bodyplanstarter

2. Bathroom scales

A *Body Fat* reading on your scales is preferable but not compulsory. I will go into detail further in *Chapter 3: Keeping Records* on how much importance to place on the *body fat* result.

3. Tape measure

4. Tripod for your smartphone to take progress photos

Alternatively, you can ask a loved one to take these photos or prop your camera/smartphone up in the same place each time.

5. Calorie counter app

Download *Lose It* or *My Fitness Pal* app to your smartphone (I personally prefer *Lose It*).

6. Digital kitchen scales

If more than one of you in the household is going to partake in *The Body Plan*, then I highly recommend you get one each to use at meal times, as they're often inexpensive. We have one for me and one for my husband.

PART I

MY PHILOSOPHY

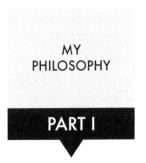

Where does a philosophy on weight loss come from? Is it purely from the books you read, the diets you follow, the 'gurus' you trust, the personal training sessions you sign up for or is it a combination of all of them? The truth is that it's all of them and none of them. Huh? Let me explain.

My decade as a flight attendant began in my mid-twenties,

where body image played a significant part in my career and lifestyle. Health and well-being not so much, as there was always a party to attend or country to fly to.

Whatever latest diet craze was fair game for me and my fellow 'flighties' as we worked through the *Quick Cleanse* detox, *Atkins* (low carb), the *South Beach* diet and Jennifer Aniston's favourite *The Zone*. Then there were the shakes and bars, and more frequently the room service steamed veggies that balanced out our in-room wine nights. I'm sure there is more, but I think you get the picture, and I bet you're also no stranger to these or similar fad diets.

And let's not forget those few years I was renowned as a raw food advocate. In 2014, Woman's Day Australia named me *Australia's Leading Raw Chef* after I formalised my keen love of raw food by training as a *Raw Food Chef* in the USA with one of the world's most recognised culinary schools.

Don't get me wrong, I still stand by many of the health benefits I advocated as a raw food educator, but at this stage in my life the philosophy is no longer practical, nor is it desirable for me to mostly eat raw fruits, vegetables, seeds and nuts.

After I left full-time work and started my family, as is usual for many new parents I really lost my way with my self-care. The transition to my new life took all my energy, and my weight continued to rise as I placed very little importance on my diet while caring for my family.

I remember a moment when I went to see my GP to get a referral to be checked for celiac disease, as half my family have it so I assumed my rapid weight gain could be for only this reason.

After receiving a negative result for celiac disease, my well-meaning but incredibly incorrect doctor gave me a rumpled photocopy of a diet that many of his nursing staff were following with success. It was a diet that some famous Filipino actress was spouting and then I was sent on my way.

I had even had my thyroid tested, seeking some form of 'medical' reason for my weight problem after having my babies. The specialist thought I'd be happy to learn that I had no issues with my thyroid, but my weight gain was purely from over-eating and being too inactive. Of course, I was half happy as I didn't want a life on thyroid medication; however, I still didn't have an answer that explained my excess weight.

When I finally hit rock bottom, as mentioned in *My Story*, I realised that the only approach to shift this unwanted weight that would work for me in the long-term was going to need to be:

- practical as a busy mother,
- pleasurable so I would stick to it,
- flexible so that I could navigate around life's inevitable disruption, and
- sustainable, so that it would see me into old age, without the yo-yo effect.

In the end, my philosophy comes from a combination of common sense, which I needed to recalibrate after years of being brainwashed with easy-come, easy-go diet plans, as well as looking to those who were succeeding with similar approaches.

I sought out inspiring women, my age or older, experts (I credit many of them throughout the book) and good old practical experience (mine and my clients.)

I wanted to know what made me lose weight, maintain weight and gain weight in scientific evidence-based reality, not a wishy-washy 'new found secret'. I just wanted the facts, so I could compile my own framework for a new way of eating that I could adhere to forever, without issue.

If you've tried and failed with many of the other 'diets' out there, then I hear you. I understand the devastation you've felt when you've regained that weight and then some, after all the hard work you've put in with restricting your food or pounding yourself in the gym.

You can believe me because I've lived it, and achieved it and continued to sustain my results, through travel, special occasions and unsettling times in mine and my family's lives. The proof is in my results.

There are a few parts to my *Philosophy*. Firstly, I'm going to smash through some commonly thought *myths;* I learnt these the hard way, so I'm going to step you through them, so you don't have to! Then I'm going to take you through the connection between the *Body*, *Mind* and *Soul*, and why none of my weight loss attempts worked until I had these three crucial parts of myself in sync.

Ready? Let's dive in with busting some *myths* first.

MYTH BUSTING

*B*efore I share the exact steps I took for my own body transformation, I'd like to share with you my personal philosophy that underpinned my body transformation. I'd also like to dispel some *myths* that might currently be holding you back from your own success.

Are you ready?

Where do these *myths* come from? Fads that pop up? Celebrities going on about their success (when they don't tell you half the story!) What your well-intentioned grandma told you? What worked for you at one point in your life (but hey if it genuinely worked why are you here?) *Myths* can be more seductive than truth, and some of them will bounce back more than common sense. What happens when you believe them? You're on a fast road to failure, and that's not where we want you to go on this journey!

Ever heard of these and thought they were true?

- "You need rock-solid discipline."
- "You have to give up your favourite foods."
- "You have to exercise like crazy."

- "You'll have to eat chicken and broccoli for
  every meal."
- "You cannot eat carbs (or 'white foods' or any other
  food group for that matter!)"
- "Dieting/losing weight means hunger."
- "Progress is best measured by the bathroom scales."
- "Intuitive eating is superior to portion control."

Think again. All of the above statements are *myths*. Let's get started with needing to have rock-solid discipline.

Myth #1 You need rock-solid discipline to achieve the kind of transformation I have been able to have

I am here to tell you 'hell no!' I love a good cupcake or three especially when I have been slaving over the oven baking them for the latest bake sale at school or for a friend's birthday. I also have been known to enjoy a delicious, crisp prosecco with friends as this is the end of the week ritual at our local rugby club while the kids are playing sport. My dinner these nights is often a yummy burger or pork belly roll. Or a random late night out with friends, watching live music or making shapes on the dance floor. I also enjoy a slice or two of pizza with the family when I can't be bothered to cook that night, or to hit up our favourite Thai hole in the wall restaurant. Not to forget that cheeky bit of chocolate just before the monthlies hit. Or the fish and chips with mushy peas at the British club, while the kids catch up with friends in the pool. One of my favourites.

You too can achieve long-lasting, sustainable weight loss and not have to give up any of your favourite foods, because let's face it, life is to be enjoyed too. I believe that if you restrict, then you increase your risk of bingeing, so if you're an all or nothing person like I have been pretty much all my life, prepare to be amazed in these following pages.

Myth #2 You have to give up your favourite foods

Nope. You can still enjoy all your favourites, even if they're considered 'unhealthy'. Not to excess mind you, but hey, nothing in excess has ever been good for us. I've gotta tell you, one of my favourite things in the world is those deliciously decadent Cadbury creme eggs. Do you think I didn't enjoy any of them at Easter time? Hell no! I had about four. Or six. I can't quite remember right now, but you know what, it didn't impact my weight loss plan at all, nor did I feel the guilts after enjoying them. Did I spend two hours on the treadmill trying to work the buggers off? Nope. I'll show you the exact way I was able to lose weight still, lose the guilt, eliminate any bingeing following restriction and still enjoy food.

Myth #3 You have to exercise like crazy

Again, this is wrong. Well for me anyway. Plenty of people will tell you that when they work out, they feel their diet is much better because intuitively they don't want to undo all the hard work they've done by pounding themselves at the gym or outdoors. I get that. I know that feeling too. But for those of you who don't much love the gym or have very little time to spare around work and family life to embark on a new fitness regime, listen up. I want to implore you to work first on your diet. You can lose weight through diet alone, but of course, there are health benefits to be had from being active. If you need to lose weight and your health depends on it, focus first on your food and diet, then the fitness can follow-up next. Hitting the gym doesn't need to be an every day thing. I'll talk about this later in the book.

Myth #4 You'll have to eat chicken and broccoli for every meal

I'll admit, when I first started on my journey, I was eating bucket loads of chicken and broccoli, and often it's my fall back for a simple healthy and filling meal. But it's not all you have to eat.

Jeff Cavaliere, one of my husband's favourite *YouTube* personalities for fitness and health, says that when it comes to diet, we all have these choices to make:

- *fast*
- *cheap, or*
- *good (healthy).*

According to him, we can achieve only two of the three, and we can't get all three at once.

To apply *fast* and *cheap*, I might opt to bulk grill loads of chicken breast (or any other lean protein for that matter) and prepare my vegetables ahead of time so that we can have quick and affordable meals ready for those days we have limited time for meal preparation in our household. But for the other times when I have more time to spend on making more varied meals, I might be able to make *good* (healthy) meals that are affordable with prior planning and farmer's market trips. On the flip side, when you need something that's *fast* and *cheap*, it's quite often going to be a poor nutritional choice (drive-thru anyone?)

When you become more confident with how to plan your meals out, and what your daily budget spend is, which I talk more about further in the book, then you will realise there are some really delicious options to be had. Plus, nothing is disallowed. This really blew my friend's mind when I sent her a photo of my hangover cure one day; a plate of nachos that I'd made myself after a big night out. She couldn't comprehend my 'diet' would allow it and told me that it was not bodybuilder food. Ha, I showed her!

Myth #5 You cannot eat carbs (or insert another food group here)

This is one myth I adore dispelling. We've all been there. On the low carb/no-carb diet, where a McDonald's burger was acceptable as long as you didn't eat the bun. Or don't even think about an apple. And as long as your pee on the stick showed you were in ketosis, you could drink as much cream in your coffee as you desired. Oh my God, I've never craved a banana or a piece of bread so much in my life.

And how many times have you tried to be 'good' by eliminating some kind of food you really enjoy, like the delicious sourdough bread with butter, or that homemade cookie only to desire it even more (and likely end up stuffing your face with it when it was next available!)

A study done at *University of Montreal's* Faculty of Medicine found that a diet high in fat and sugary foods can cause chemical changes in the brain so that when these are removed the withdrawal feelings can be as severe as drug withdrawal and cause sensitivity to stress and anxiety, sometimes even depression. This, in turn, can create a rebound effect: a return to eating those high-fat and sugary foods.

So why not include a little of those foods to keep the stress, anxiety and depression at bay. I'll show you how you can.

Myth #6 Dieting/losing weight means insatiable hunger

It's a common myth that to lose weight you must be in a state of restriction and denial and I want to share with you that during the entire time of my journey I have never felt so free and empowered, which is the opposite to denial right? Of course, to experience the changes you want, you are going to need to make some adaptations to the way you currently eat and live. You might just find however that with just a few tweaks you aren't going to feel like eating your arm off.

With some of my coaching clients, when we first looked at their current eating habits and then modified them, many of them couldn't believe how much more food they were eating. In fact, some of them struggled to even eat that amount.

It's entirely possible that with your current food choices you may be under-eating or even not getting enough nutrients as well if you never feel hungry. It's all perspective. If you're not eating the best quality of food, you may be under-consuming in some areas and over-eating in others. When you get a better take on your new and improved lifestyle, it's likely you're not going to feel hunger, and if you're carrying extra unwanted weight, it will start to fall off.

Myth #7 Progress is best measured by the bathroom scales

Weighing yourself is only giving you a part of the picture. If you're solely relying on those little digits to be going down each time you weigh yourself to show you're making progress, you're bound to be disappointed. Throughout six-months, my weight fluctuated within the same range of two to three kilograms; however, my measurements continued to decline consistently in a downward trend. This indicating that even though my weight wasn't so much shifting at times, my body was getting smaller through what is known as re-composition. This is because my body was reducing body fat while building lean muscle.

Myth #8 Intuitive eating is superior to portion control

Intuitive eating sounds terrific in theory. It's something I have been getting closer to achieving through *The Body Plan* and described in further detail in this book. But I do fear that using intuitive eating as a weight-control mode can be what holds many people back from having the success they desire. Relying purely on your intuition to portion control, which is quite possibly broken through a life of excess, busy living, detachment to what you eat or even misinterpretation of hunger signals, may not yield you the desired results you seek.

In my personal experience and after discussions with experts (personal trainers, nutritionists and others in the industry working with real-life clients), those that do succeed with intuitive eating to maintain their lean healthy weight or are using it as a tool to achieve their dream body, have already done some form of self-awareness or data collection. Perhaps like logging of food intake or management in the past to get to know their own personal needs and understand true and honest portion control.

I've had a few days here and there where I haven't ended up logging or consciously managing my food intake, however subconsciously I've been able to stick to a similar food intake because I've reached a better level of understanding my body. My hunger cues, my satisfaction levels and how different types and volumes of food make me feel.

In contrast, before I started this plan, even with my extensive nutritional knowledge and background, I thought my intuitive eating was enough to keep me lean and healthy.

But it wasn't, and ultimately my lack of understanding and self-awareness contributed to my weight gain after I'd finished pregnancy and nursing my children.

Even though it appeared I was eating what's considered

healthful foods, no matter how you slice it, if you are eating more energy than your body needs, where do you think it's going to go? You are going to store it as fat.

And what's funny is, I didn't even think I was eating a great deal of food, but I wasn't eating consistently nor was I also mindful of the kinds of foods I was eating from day-to-day. Which is common as many of us prioritise everything else; family, work, school, friends etc., just relying on the next meal showing up.

Robyn's recommendation

Open your mind and cast aside those limiting beliefs and restrictive behaviours that you've relied on in the past but unsuccessful weight loss attempts. Realise that there are many, varied and flexible ways to attack your goal. Before we move further into the book, understand there is no one approach, fad diet, system or theory that works in isolation. Following a guru simply just doesn't work. Know what works for you and then create a plan that is an amalgam of things you believe. There is no black or white solution, no magic pill. And everything in the marketplace is open to interpretation and often designed to rid you of your hard-earned cash, not just your fat.

BODY

When you want or need to lose fat, for your health, the only way you are going to achieve it is by creating a *calorie deficit*.

A *calorie deficit* essentially means you consume fewer calories (energy) than your body needs, therefore enabling a shortfall in calories or energy consumption. This will become clearer in *Chapter 4: Understanding Flexible Dieting.*

That's it. Simple right?

You don't need to buy into the latest diet fad to achieve your goals. However, the reason they do work is that you are creating a calorie deficit.

- The *ketogenic* diet works, when you're in a calorie deficit.
- The *raw vegan* diet works, when you're in a calorie deficit.
- The *juicing* diet works, when you're in a calorie deficit.
- The *paleo* diet works, when you're in a calorie deficit.

- The *meal replacement shake* diet works, when you're in a calorie deficit.
- The *intermittent fasting* diet works, when you're in a calorie deficit.

So, what do we need to cover to make calories work for you and not against you?

- The importance of keeping accurate records
- Remove fitness as the focus
- Focus on your own plate
- Apply the 70/20/10 Rule, and
- Manage your environment

So, let's get started with understanding the importance of good record keeping.

The importance of keeping accurate records

What I've discovered on my own journey was the value in record keeping and data collection. Now don't get me wrong. I am married to the spreadsheet king, and he does tend to take it a little far at times, but if there is one thing he and I agree on, it's keeping as much data as possible as you progress through your journey. This will help you to build and understand your own unique situation. The more information you can collect, the better your appreciation of where you're at and how to move forward, each step of the way.

When you first start out, because it's unlikely you've been collecting the kind of data you'll need for this game plan, you will be creating a baseline created by standardised scientific biological formulas to begin with, to give you an estimated individual starting point.

Because of this, your own personal weekly targets will require refining as time goes by. This is why it's ever so important for you to record not only your weight but also your measurements and photos, as well as your food intake, so you can audit your progress and make refinements as the weeks go by.

I'll show you what to do in *Part II, Chapter 3: Keeping Records.*

Remove fitness as the focus

What is one of the first things most people do when they feel they need to lose some weight?

They start a new fitness routine.

Because exercise is how you lose weight right?

Yes and no.

Four weeks after a normal and healthy delivery with my second child, I was given the go-ahead to resume my usual exercise regime of spin classes, boot camps and weight training on the compound I was living in, in Saudi Arabia.

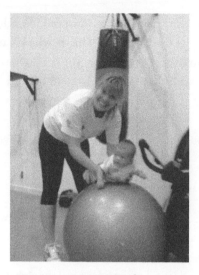

Saudi Arabia, 2013

And from this moment on, after my initial and immediate post labour weight loss, my weight steadily began to climb up to my highest weight ever, three years later. This was when I finally decided to do something serious about it: I outline the plan in this book.

Even in the months before me starting this particular game plan, I was training way harder than I had in these last eighteen months of my body transformation. I even thought a self-imposed thirty consecutive days of spin class challenge would shift some kilograms, but it didn't at all. In fact, it made me eat more, which set me back in my fat loss goals.

Ever heard these?

"You can't outrun a bad diet."

or

"Abs are made in the kitchen."

It's true! Fitness has its place in a healthy lifestyle, but not when you are just beginning your weight loss journey. This is when fitness can be counterproductive. Often people will train then eat back their calories earned and then some.

In *Secrets From the Eating Lab: The Science of Weight Loss, the Myth of Willpower and Why You Should Never Diet Again,* Traci Mann PhD says that exercise doesn't typically lead to dramatic weight loss.

One of the main reasons it doesn't work as well as we'd love it to is because it takes way too much exercise to work off that cookie (or three) we had with our morning coffee.

Susan Peirce Thompson, PhD of *Bright Line Eating: The Science of Living Happy, Thin & Free,* also advocates a low or no exercise regime when you are in weight-loss mode. She says not only does the energy expenditure you consume in one sitting far exceed what you could burn off in a morning at the gym, but over time of regular exercise, your body starts to demand more food, and so you compensate your higher activity levels by eating more, which is counterproductive to weight loss.

If you've had success with weight loss in the past when you have been exercising, the success occurred because you also made dietary changes at the same time. This is common when we make a conscious act to start working out. Some of us find it more encouraging to stick to a healthier diet when knowing how hard we trained at the gym that day, but it's not always the case, as studies have proven that exercise can reduce self-control too.

This doesn't mean you should never exercise again, but I want you to take it off the table for at least the next month or three while you focus on getting your nutrition on point.

You'll understand as you progress further in the book why it's important to minimise your decision making and tasks while in this crucial stage of honing and automating your eating habits.

The beauty of taking fitness off the table for the first one to three months is you'll also free up extra time to devote to learning, meal preparation and effective habit-stacking.

Just like learning a new language or how to play an instrument or new sport takes time to finesse, you really owe yourself the time to master and implement these new (or maybe not so new) diet and nutrition tweaks. Then they will become habitual and instinctual. Everything that is a departure from the norm for you will become progressively more natural over time.

So when should we exercise? Exercise is most definitely an essential component of a healthy lifestyle, so please do not mistake my intentions. If you already incorporate movement or some form of intentional exercise into your regime then, by all means, please don't stop with the introduction to what I share here.

My intention here is to merely give you permission for the next three months to not overdo the lifestyle changes, so that you end up ultimately doing none, and continue along the path you are already on, a path of dissatisfaction.

If you are already attending regular yoga classes, or a long brisk walk after dinner (or before work for that matter) or an enjoyable dance class with friends, or nothing at all. Change nothing, until you feel comfortable with your new eating habits.

If you get to the point where you have to choose between meal planning or hitting the gym, always choose to manage your food as a priority first. Until it all becomes quite natural and efficient. Then you can re-introduce the fitness aspect. I will share more of my own fitness journey in my follow-up book, as this was not a focus for me during the first three months.

Exercise helps with lung and heart health, libido and so much more. I really don't want to go into too much detail about it here as it's not something I'm an expert on, and it didn't become a priority for me until after three months.

If you are keen to get into your exercise and know without a doubt you can manage it and a change in your eating habits, then my advice to you is this:

- Simplify your exercise.
- Don't overcomplicate it.
- Stop overthinking it.
- Find something you enjoy and do it consistently.

This will allow you to develop a love for more complicated training organically over time.

"The real benefits of exercise come with months and years of sustained, steady growth. Short-term gains in fitness are fun but misleading" according to Henry S. Lodge M.D. from *Younger Next Year for Women: Live Strong, Fit, and Sexy—Until You're 80 and Beyond.*

So, give yourself time and space to build up to it and to grow into a fitness program that is going to serve you well into your eighties and beyond.

Focus on the input first (what you eat), not output (exercise and movement) because the feedback technology to accurately determine how much you are burning off just doesn't exist. Whatever your calorie watch/tracker on your wrist says is very subjective and not reliable, so don't rely on it for 'earning back' your calories.

Focus on your own plate

One of the hardest things to do when you first start making radical changes to the way you eat and move, especially if you're the primary caregiver of your family, is how to get everyone else in your home on board.

Well here's my secret.

You don't.

Not at first anyway. The reason being, if this is such a brand-new practice for you to learn and apply, you don't need the added pressure of trying to make it fit everyone else's needs in the household at the same time, or else that's just not going to work.

That's not to say that it won't eventually end up that way and that you don't want to fuel your family in the same healthful ways that you are going to be looking after yourself, but it will come. I promise. Leading by example is one such way to inspire them with your healthy changes.

Just like in my good old days as a flight attendant, it's time to put your own oxygen mask on first, so then you can help others afterwards.

It may seem like more work, different meals for everyone, but hear me out. I will share with you further in the book about how I've managed to do this as stress-free as possible.

And if you're concerned about trying to change and improve your families eating and health habits as well, if they need it, then why not be the pioneer. As most of us already know, quietly setting the example first rather than telling family members to try something new, can often yield more significant results.

The 70 / 20 / 10 rule

How many times have you heard or said to yourself 'tomorrow I'll be good' or 'after my holidays I'll be back on the wagon' or something similar?

The thing with these 'diets' that you've tried in the past and failed on is they don't allow you any wiggle room so that the minute you indulge in your favourite pre-monthly chocolate, it rapidly turns into the whole bar. Or you have a post-hangover fry up, and you feel like the biggest failure ever.

Well, newsflash lady! This is real life.

Unless you're moving to a remote little village in the middle of nowhere, where you have to grow your own food and you have no friends, or don't celebrate birthdays or have work lunches and farewells, then you have to adapt to a system that works in the real world.

I love food, and if I had to deny myself some of my favourite and most pleasurable meals, then I'd give up right away.

Life is to be enjoyed whether it's your kid's birthday cake, or indulging in some local cuisine on holiday, you have to make this work for you, in a way that you will stick to throughout your life.

That means making nothing off limits. Of course, I'm not referring to severe food allergies or diseases. You need to discuss these with your medical provider, but when it comes to enjoying a treat here and there, go for it.

So how do I manage it?

You may have heard of the 80 / 20 rule?

Well, I follow the 70 / 20 / 10 rule, which is based on nutrition researcher and educator, Alan Aragon's *10 Essential Characteristics of a Balanced Diet*. His looks similar to my own adaptation which I created to suit me. I talk more about his definition of a balanced diet in *Chapter 4: Understanding Flexible Dieting.*

Seventy per cent of my daily intake consists of unprocessed whole food ingredients, the best quality I can afford. Do I always buy organic? Hell no! As much as I wish I could, it's just not practical for my family and me, but we do our best where we can. These categories of foods are things like fresh eggs, fresh farm vegetables, and fruits, lean meats like chicken and local fish. Basically, foods that haven't been tampered with or they've been handled very little by humans or machines.

Twenty per cent of my daily diet allows for questionable healthy foods. These are foods that are often labelled as healthy and have been processed to some degree. These could be cheeses and yoghurts, oats, pasta, rice, sauces and flavourings, low/no-calorie sweeteners, dark chocolate, nut butter. These are still considered relatively healthy to eat in smaller amounts, but they have been processed in some form or another and are not as natural as the previous whole foods category.

And of course, 10 per cent pure junk. Why not? Junk food has been created to be desirable, tastes good and usually pretty appealing which makes it hard for the majority of the human race to resist. These could be things like French fries, pizza, alcohol, birthday cake etc.

To deny yourself completely from enjoying any of these foods would be almost impossible to resist forever in the world we live in today, and quite often results in desiring it way more than you would if you had just allowed yourself a small amount.

Sure, common sense tells us that it's not a great idea to eat a diet that is a 100 per cent junk food oriented but enjoying guilty pleasures in small moderation is actually more virtuous that 80 per cent of the Western population, which is currently consuming 40 per cent plus of a diet high in processed foods.

Manage your environment

You are the average of the people you surround yourself with. There are just some things you cannot change, like genetics, health history, energy levels, cravings, but you can manipulate other factors: the type of food you keep in your house, people to spend time with, the way you spend your leisure time and the way you prepare your meals ahead of time. Dedicate your time to creating a nurturing environment that will align with your goals. I'll go into more detail as to how to do this in *Chapter 2: Creating the Space & Clearing the Chaos.*

Robyn's recommendation

Stop focusing on fitness as a fat loss solution and concentrate entirely on nutrition and your lifestyle habits for the first three months. Do not start any new exercise program. However, if it feels comfortable to you to continue any current exercise you already have in place, by all means, keep doing it, but be conscious of your eating habits first and foremost during this time.

Work hard on your environment. Be conscious of the people you spend the most time with or are around and modify your environment if necessary or possible. Ideally be around people who are in better shape than you, both mentally and physically. This will help to inspire you. Work out with them (just don't focus on this aspect in the first three months). Be around people whom you wish to be like. If this is not practical in real life, then find people online that you resonate with (*YouTube, Instagram or Facebook* groups) to keep your inspiration at a high level. Not everyone in your social circle is going to be where you ideally want to be, but try to skew it in the direction of the more positive.

MIND

Your inner transformation needs to occur before your outer one.

So, what am I referring to when I talk about *Mind*? It's about controlling the monkey mind that dictates what we do with our *body* and *soul*. It's how we think, how our thoughts affect our actions and if you're not in control of it, what will run you off your road to weight loss success and healthy lifestyle management! When we talk about getting the *mind* under control, we need to address the following things:

- understanding the importance of your mindset,
- accepting delayed gratification,
- eliminating timelines,
- breaking your current cycle,
- recognising why willpower won't work,
- avoiding decision fatigue,

- building new habits through automation and repetition,
- practising the arts of habit-stacking and kedging, and
- becoming relentless.

Shall we start with the first beast, taming your established perspective, *your mindset?*

Your mindset

Before even considering the methods I used to lose weight, it's essential that you realise the physical change is not going to happen without you committing to doing the inner work first. Especially if you desire long-term success. It's crucial not to overlook this mindset stuff, as it will really help you hit your goal and stay there for years to come.

I'm convinced you don't intend to be another statistic of dieters that return to their pre-dieting weight and habits, so doing this groundwork is imperative for your success.

According to Gary Foster, Ph.D., clinical director of the *Weight and Eating Disorders Program* at the *University of Pennsylvania*, nearly 65 per cent of dieters return to their pre-diet weight within three years.

Before the outside results can appear, you need to be committed to the internal transformation first. Your dedication to your inner self will eventually show up on the outside as you get leaner and healthier.

When I refer to this internal work, what I am really meaning is the collective: mental health, beliefs, mindset, emotional needs, anything that relates to the way you feel and the way you think. This can also refer to spirituality, soul, your purpose or meaning of life which I discuss more in the following section, *Soul.*

The most significant change with my own body transformation hasn't been in the way my body looks or performs, it's been in working on creating a new and improved mindset and way of thinking.

As someone that has always been a go-getter and results driven, previously not stopping until hitting my goal or burn out, whichever came first, I've recently discovered the value of patience and kindness to oneself.

When you change your *mind*, you effectively change your life. But at first, it may not seem that simple.

According to Dr Joe Dispenza, author of *Breaking the Habit of Being Yourself: How to Lose Your Mind and Create a New One*, trying to change your emotional pattern can be like going through drug withdrawal, as change requires new ways of thinking, doing and being.

He also teaches that once you change your internal state, you no longer need the external world to give you a reason to feel happiness, gratitude or other positive emotions because, at that moment, your physical body feels it as if it is experiencing it right now.

These high emotions will help you to move into a state of being where your desire will feel as if it has already happened thereby taking you closer towards it in reality.

Before you can experience a new event, you need first to think it, feel it and then be it.

Giving me permission to realise this was not going to be an overnight change and that I was in this for the long-haul was also the most significant transformation of all.

Have unwavering faith that you can create the body of your dreams. It is possible. You just need to have the vision and the commitment to that vision.

Delayed gratification

I need you to sit down for the following section because it's likely to be unpleasant for you to read.

Drop the need and desire for instant gratification.

This transformation is not going to be a quick and easy fix, but it will be worth it.

If you're carrying considerable excess weight, I'm afraid you're not going to get your bikini body in time for your vacation in six weeks. Or else if you do, it's likely you're going to rebound even worse when you return to healthy eating because to have achieved it, you've had to do something pretty radical that is unlikely to be sustainable for you moving forward.

When I accepted that any long-lasting change would require some significant modifications to my beliefs, internal dialogue, mental, emotional and possibly even spiritual health, was when I knew I would finally have the weight loss I dreamed of. New habits and behaviour needed to be developed that would be sustainable and last forever.

A younger friend of mine, in her late twenties, who I had recently met after I'd lost the majority of my weight, wanted to know how long it had taken me and what I had done to do it. Naturally, as I've written this book to describe in detail what I have done, a short answer was all that I could give her. Knowing her current 'restrict then over-eat' habits weren't getting her any closer to her goals, I merely told her that I had been on this path two years and I was still going.

She then told me she didn't have two years. She wanted results sooner than that.

Listen, I get that need. Two years seems so far away, and you've got that holiday coming up in two months. But what if you kept trying with what you've currently been doing (or not doing) and two years later you were still in the same position. Or worse, you'd gained even more weight and frustration.

And what twenty-something doesn't have two years. With any luck, we're all going to be around for quite some time. Even me, aged 38, gave it a good crack for two years, and even within three months I was already feeling the positive effects of my new lifestyle habits.

The way I see it you have three choices to make:

1. Don't change anything and two years will arrive, and you will have gained more weight. Recent studies have shown that adults' weights are increasing by approximately 500g – 1kg per year,
2. Attempt one or many fad diets, that promise you quick results, that may deliver immediate results for an event or holiday, but after restricting before then over-eating afterwards, you'll be right back where you started, or even fatter, or
3. Make peace with slow, manageable, sustainable and successful weight loss that will have a continuing trend of always going down until you hit your goal. This is primarily the philosophy that this book and plan is founded upon.

Remind yourself that with any luck, with the beauty of this gift we call life, you'll be here for a good while yet. That the next twelve months are going to pass by whether you make these positive lifestyle enhancements or not. So why not look back in a year knowing that you took inspired action and made a positive change for yourself, for the better. You'll wish you'd started sooner!

If you look at many of the world's wealthiest and most

successful people, many of them have remained vigilant and laser-focused on their long-term vision. They've been able to forgo the short-term solution in favour of a longer-term desired outcome.

Have you heard of *The Stanford Marshmallow Experiment?* It was a series of studies on delayed gratification in the late 1960s and early 1970s led by psychologist Walter Mischel.

Preschool children were given an option, either eat the marshmallow now or wait an indeterminable amount of time and they could eat two marshmallows.

The idea being you can have a smaller reward up front or a bigger bonus if you wait.

I'm sure we all remember back to our childhood days when our parents tried to teach us the value of saving our pocket money rather than spending it on candy or toys, something we might do with our own children now.

I won't deny we haven't tried our own version of the marshmallow experiment in our own household with our kids.

In a follow-up study, it was found that those children who delayed their own gratification in the original survey were proven to be more competent as adolescents with higher SAT scores at high school.

We don't need this kind of experiment to highlight what we already know about delayed gratification, but it's hard to remain on course when we're bombarded with advertising and marketing wherever we look for the latest quick fix.

I'll never forget my grandparents telling me that when they first married and started their family, they would save up for each piece of furniture or large cost item they needed, not buying anything until they could buy it outright. If they couldn't pay cash, they wouldn't buy it.

When was the last time you used your credit card to make a purchase? Or bought a large appliance on interest-free.

We are a society that lives on credit; we desire immediate solutions to our problems and continuously need to be stimulated. I'm not convinced this is progression, but that's probably a whole new book in itself.

When I first set out on my body transformation, ten months before I hit forty, I intended to reach my ultimate goal weight by my birthday. But I also wanted to ensure a sustainable process, that would be pleasurable and not punishment.

As my birthday loomed, I made peace with potentially not reaching the ultimate goal I initially set out for myself, but it didn't come naturally. It did take some severe inner self-talk to accept because we've been conditioned as a society to strive for and accept quick solutions to our problems.

During this acceptance process, I realised a few months short of my birthday, having been on my transformation for seven months or so, I had already achieved so much. I had created new habits and learnt so much more about myself, and my capabilities. That is equal to, if not greater than the end result, in my opinion, as these habits will continue long after I've hit my target and sustain me into old age, I hope.

In a society that promises quick fixes and short-term results, it's sometimes a challenge to come to terms with this, but genuinely knowing and trusting that I want to be here for a long time, not just a good time, has helped me to drop the short-term mindset.

One hour times twenty-four hours makes a day, one day times seven adds up to a week and four weeks make a month. Time never stops and will pass by regardless of how you chose to spend your time. You get the picture.

That time is going to pass you by no matter what you do with it, so don't sit back and be a passenger on the sidelines of your life. Take control of the wheel.

Eliminate timelines

This transformation is going to take time. And the length of time for me may be different for you. This required a little extra inner work for me to realise and accept, especially in a society that values fast results. I had to remind myself that I could hit my goal in record time, but needed to consider what sacrifice would it take for me to get there and would it be sustainable and long-lasting. These were both valuable to me, not just hitting my goal.

I recall a moment at the Rugby club one evening when I met a man who had been on his own weight loss journey for as long as I had, with apparently fewer sacrifices that I had seemingly made, announcing that he was able to have lost his weight while still enjoying a few beers each night. He claimed he did no exercise and had lost way more weight than I had in the same period. That was enough to send me spiralling into a night of a few too many drinks and pork rolls, upset with myself that it was taking me longer to achieve, with what I felt were more compensations.

In the end, I had to realise this is a very personal and unique journey and who knows what his own history was and if he was likely to keep the weight off once he returned to his previous habits.

I had to keep my eyes in my own lane and be confident that I was building compounding habits that I was not going to return from, that were achievable in my own life, and were going to produce results for life.

I later discovered this guy was eating from a calorie-controlled meal service, didn't have children nor those responsibilities that came with parenthood. He had started at a much larger weight than I, had a completely different lifestyle to me and wasn't actually learning any skills that he could use once he stopped the meal service. Each to their own, but after I got over my hangover and recovery from that night out, I was able to see that this was my journey and that it would take however long it needed to and to also appreciate how far I had already come. His results were irrelevant to me and my own path.

Breaking the cycle

I totally get how difficult it is to break a cycle or change your usual habits, because often you've been operating the same way for quite some time, to the point that you don't even think about it.

According to an article on lifehack.org, Eugene K. Choi, the founder of *Destiny Hacks*, a blog and coaching service; *"About 40 per cent of the things you do in a day doesn't involve you actively making a decision. Instead, it is actually a habit."* This sounds about right if you are truly honest about the tasks you perform throughout a day.

So, the key is to put in a little effort in the beginning to create a habit that will eventually become such second nature that you don't even need to think about it.

A great example of how I have applied this is that I never used to eat breakfast, and would only start eating during the day when my tummy demanded it, usually lunch time to mid-afternoon.

Then of course when I really felt the hunger kick in, I would grab whatever was nearest or most convenient to me. Often it was processed or not mindful. Or scraps off the kids' plates. I know you've done it too.

Since then, I've automated my meal times by eating at roughly the same time every day, and often the same kinds of foods. Every morning as soon as I hit the kitchen to prepare school lunch boxes, the oats go directly into the *thermomix* to make my breakfast without me even having to decide "what do I feel like today?" It's just like brushing my teeth which I don't even think about.

I tend to rotate the same eight to ten main meals each week and I mostly bulk prepare them, so when it comes to my set meal times, there is no thinking required.

You'll find that people who've been regularly physically active for an extended period, whether it be as a runner, gym bunny or any other kind of activity say the same. They've been doing it so long now, they don't even question why they do it. They just pop on their shoes, rain, hail or shine and go through the motions.

Willpower won't work

Conventional diets require you to resist certain foods, not just once, but over and over again. The first or second time you refuse might be a success, but after you've been saying 'no' throughout a day, your willpower will be tested.

Willpower is like your smartphone battery. It's a finite resource, and once you've been using it all day, it begins to run low to almost non-existent, until you replenish it again, which usually happens overnight as you sleep.

As Traci Mann Ph.D from *Secrets from the Eating Lab* says, *"Humans were simply not made to will-fully resist food. We evolved through famines, hunting, and gathering, eating whatever we could get when we could get it. We evolved to keep fat on our bones by eating the foods that we see, not resisting them. It is difficult to imagine how any species could evolve to be successful at resisting the foods that keep it alive."*

It's not because you lack discipline or have no willpower compared to that naturally thin friend of yours. It's because you're human.

Things that deplete your willpower reserves:

- making decisions,
- multi-tasking, and
- trying to be in control of more than one thing simultaneously.

Relying on willpower to have long-term success is a failed approach and ultimately will be the kiss of death.

Learning how to not lean on self-control to have the weight loss success you desire will make the whole unfolding of your body transformation pleasant and sustainable for a long time to come.

Decision fatigue

Decision fatigue occurs when you've been making cumulative and essential decisions throughout the day which in turn depletes your willpower battery. This means any further decisions you're likely to make that day do not get the full attention they deserve, and you begin to experience mental slowdown or tiredness.

This has been proven in a study on judicial rulings http://www.pnas.org/content/pnas/108/17/6889.full.pdf

Even though judges are required to hold legal reason to their cases, it was shown that more favourable rulings are apparent at the beginning of the day as opposed to later in the day. Perhaps this is due to mental fatigue from a heavy decision load.

This can show up in your own life, by having multiple essential decisions at work or at home, so that during the evening instead of making a decision on what healthy meal to cook up and hit the gym, you choose to order in pizza, relax on the couch and watch *Netflix*.

So, what's the solution, instead of relying on your willpower? Let me show you.

Building new habits through automation and repetition

A simple way to eliminate or reduce your decision making or to preserve your willpower reserves is to automate as many as possible of the repeatable tasks that you do most days, so they become habits.

You can eliminate decision fatigue by reducing the volume of decisions you need to make throughout the day by automating the most commonly occurring tasks.

For example:

- What will I have for breakfast?
- What will I wear today?
- What time will I go to the gym?
- What tasks do I need to do before going to bed?

Master a daily routine: have your clothes set out the night before going to bed, plan ahead of time precisely what to eat for each meal tomorrow by writing it in your journal or your calorie tracker ahead of time.

Meal plan and prepare in bulk during your weekends or a day that you can set aside during the week.

Other ways to overcome this decision fatigue or replenish your stores is to have a rest or a disruptor like going outdoors in nature for a walk or meditation. Do something to improve your mood or increase glucose levels in the body (eat something as long as it fits your budget for the day which you will learn more about in *Chapter 4: Understanding Flexible Dieting*).

Habit-stacking

Habit-stacking is the practice of slowly introducing smaller more desirable behaviours with a larger goal in mind. The idea is that these bite-sized habits, when introduced incrementally over time, become part of your regular routine with little to no stress. You master the first habit before 'stacking' the next new habit you need to take you closer to your goal.

By introducing these habits slowly and with a strategy, you are less likely to become overwhelmed, stressed or resistant to the change.

Focus on small, daily actions that compound on each other for your overall, more significant outcome, rather than trying to change everything all at once. You will hopefully have another thirty to forty years ahead, so what is a year or two out of your life in the bigger scheme of things? Why do we only ever focus on rapid results?

When we're ready to make a change, usually something is motivating us. And when we're motivated, we tend to run at our goals full speed. We want to take action and achieve results now.

Building new, long-lasting habits can be challenging, especially if these new habits you desire are vastly different from where you currently reside.

To truly experience the most impact, I urge you to take this habit change part seriously.

The more habits you try to change all at the same time, the less chance you have of them remaining for the rest of your life, which is what we're aiming for here.

Focus on making small improvements, doing better this week than last week, so that your changes, no matter how small, compound on each other and cumulate to your desired result over time.

Be intentional and focused on the one habit until you master it and it becomes so automatic that you no longer need to think about doing it. Then add in your next and follow the same process.

What does this look like in real life?

Applying this approach of habit-stacking to your own transformation might look like this, mastering each habit below before moving onto the next:

1. Reduce your calorie intake, then
2. Reduce your consumption of processed/packaged foods, then
3. Go to bed earlier, then
4. Learn three new main meals, then
5. Begin or increase your current activity level, then
6. Limit alcohol to one night per week, then
7. Introduce weight training, then
8. Walk more, drive less.

This is just an example of how you could structure your own habit stack, to make your transformation more manageable and enjoyable.

Kedging

If life feels a little full for you at the moment or you are feeling extremely overwhelmed or 'maxed' out, your health is quite often the first thing to drop to the bottom of the priorities list.

As women, especially those with children, we've got a great knack for dropping the less critical priorities for the most, but often we neglect 'ourselves' in the cull.

Most of us are intelligent enough to know that when we don't look after ourselves over the long-term, we will burn out, get sick or somehow end up incapacitated and therefore unable to nurture those around us, or go to work, or do the many other things that have taken up the highest priority on the list. But knowing and doing are two different things.

It often takes a tragedy or illness for us to reach the point where we just have to make the change or else.

I don't want you to have to reach that point before taking action. Prevention is better than cure, but if we don't have that tragedy or misfortune to motivate us, what can we do instead?

Chris Cowley, in his book *Younger Next Year for Women: Live Strong, Fit and Sexy - Until You're 80 and Beyond*, discusses his theory on *kedging*.

Kedging is an old naval term, where boats would have a smaller boat that takes a light anchor in the direction of their destination, but not as far, and then would drop the anchor. Those on the bigger ship, once the anchor is secure, pull like crazy to drag their boat to the anchor, then it begins all over again.

So, in our circumstances, we can translate our own *kedging* or cycles (mini-milestones) to setting a goal or a focus and work like crazy to hit that goal. For me, it's been natural to place my kedges at twelve weeks and have the reward at the end – preferably something that won't undo all the good results that I've achieved, like a non-food reward.

One of my *kedges* or rewards in 2017 was going on a week-long child-free (thanks to loving grandparents and aunties) birthday trip with my hubby to Bali to celebrate my fortieth birthday.

On those days that I just didn't feel like I could face the gym (they get fewer as time goes by, believe me, and something I cover in more detail in my following book), I remembered my *kedge* or mini goal.

Another *kedge* I like to have is the promise of a new wardrobe when I hit my mini goal or a special new outfit.

Examples of other *kedges* you might like too, have been a

girls' trip away, a new piece of sporting equipment, a special event, a piece of technology or something you've been wanting for a while but been putting off.

Be relentless

Be relentless in the pursuit of your goals.

This needs to be at the forefront of anything you wish to change; don't let anything get in your way.

A friend of mine was often having weight-related injuries or ailments and was frequently talking about different health modalities she'd been exploring to get to the bottom of her inability to lose weight.

As a single woman, her weekdays were filled with work, and she lived for her weekends where she valued her social life and dance clubs.

Her best intentions to eat appropriately would often fail, as she'd prioritise her social life over grocery shopping and meal preparation, and as a single working woman, she ended up eating out most weeknights or ordering in take away.

When I suggested setting aside half a day on the weekend to bulk meal prep and plan to help ensure she was eating in alignment with her health goals, she just couldn't work out how she'd have the time.

She preferred to prioritise her social life all weekend. Her desire to make the change was not significant enough for her to take action. Your thirst for the change needs to be higher than your desire to stay the same.

Robyn's recommendations

Get excited about this process, because if you don't, it's not going to happen.

Do what you need to do to get excited.

Visualise your end result, make it fun, happy and motivating.

Select the foods you enjoy.

Don't overcomplicate it.

Not every day is going to be amazing but get excited about the journey.

Do whatever it takes to fall in love with the process, because this is a lifestyle, not a short-term plan.

Get rid of timelines and instant gratification. You need to change your relationship with food, and that is going to take more than a twelve-week program. Weight loss is not linear. Some weeks you will drop one to two kilos, and other weeks you won't lose a thing. This is normal. It's also when most people give up, but it's all part of the process. Don't have any numbers in mind because it just doesn't happen that way. Your goal is to make fitness and eating correctly a long-term lifestyle, and that takes time and consistency. This will take a while to get right. Be kind to you.

SOUL

*W*hat do I mean when I refer to *Soul*? Is it religious? Spiritual? How is it different from the *mind*?

Where in *Mind*, I cover part of my approach that is rooted in the intellectual, here in *Soul*; I discuss those aspects of *My Philosophy* that are more in line with emotions or feelings. These comprise part of our spirit as such.

I'm going to discuss:

- recognising that self-love is #1,
- getting familiar with '*Acceptance*',
- keeping your plan quiet – initially,
- knowing your core values,
- focusing on the feeling, and
- getting comfortable in '*The Waiting Room*'.

So, let's get started with recognising that self-love is actually the most crucial *soul* priority there is.

Self-love

Making the commitment to yourself to improve your health and well-being is one of the greatest acts of self-love you can do, in my opinion.

It's a misconception that wanting to improve your physical well-being is vain and obsessive, but what if we chose to look at it from the holistic point of view.

Loads of people out there will bang on about learning to love the skin you're in and loving you, as you are, right now. They may say you shouldn't need to count calories or get fixated about what you look like if you truly love who you are.

According to me, they're only half right. Why should self-improvement come at the expense of self-love? They do not need to be mutually exclusive.

Part of my own transformation required plenty of self-love and acceptance development especially as I realised my own mortality. Not just with my personal weight gain but also experiencing my ageing and achy body, the appearance of grey hairs and extra wrinkles. Add to this the environmental clues that life is finite with friends and family passing and parents growing older, etc.

I feel the greatest gift to myself and to prove my own self-love, is to work on a higher level of health and fitness.

Being disconnected from your physical health is not only going to put you at higher risk of specific ailments and diseases, but it could put you in a nursing home prematurely and have you struggling to move around earlier in old age than should be the case.

Carrying excess weight increases your chances of:

- diabetes,
- gallbladder disease and gallstones,

- heart disease and stroke,
- gout,
- high blood pressure,
- some cancers,
- liver disease,
- osteoarthritis, and
- breathing and sleep issues such as asthma and sleep apnea (stopping breathing for short stints during sleep).

A global study that researched the proportion of overweight and obese people changing over time (according to the research a *BMI* of 25-29.9 is overweight, and thirty plus is considered obese) found the following:

- High *BMI* contributed to 4 million deaths in 2015 (95 per cent confidence interval [CI] 2.7 to 5.3), representing 7.1 per cent (95 per cent CI 4.9 to 9.6) of all deaths globally.
- High *BMI* contributed to 120 million disability-adjusted life years lost (95 per cent CI 84 to 158).
- A total of 39 per cent of the deaths and 37 per cent of the disability-adjusted life years were in people with a *BMI* of less than 30 (i.e. not obese).
- Cardiovascular disease was the leading cause of death and disability-adjusted life years with 2.7 million deaths (95 per cent CI 1.8 to 3.7) and 66.3 million disability-adjusted life years (95 per cent CI 45.3 to 88.5).
- Diabetes was the second leading cause and contributed to 0.6 million deaths (95 per cent CI 0.4 to 0.7) and 30.4 million disability-adjusted life years (95 per cent CI 21.5 to 39.9).

A healthy *BMI* of 20 to 25 in adults was associated with the lowest risk of death (the UK defines this as a healthy level). Findings are taken from the NHS website here: https://www.nhs.uk/news/obesity/being-overweight-not-just-obese-still-carries-serious-health-risks/

It's still important not to mentally punish yourself for where you are right now. I practised gratitude for all that I had at this moment in time and learned to accept all that I couldn't improve on, but also to give myself permission to make improvements to my life (both physical and non-physical) and to allow the time it would take for this to occur too.

There is no time like the present to be the healthiest version of ourselves that we can be. It is the most significant act of self-love we can ever give to ourselves.

Self-acceptance

With self-love comes acceptance of where you are right now, even if nothing changed. Before I could really move forward towards my dream body, I had to stop rejecting my current state.

My self-worth could not be attached to how my body looked on the outside, because I was committed to healing the inside first. I knew if I could address my internal health then for sure my beautiful body would end up where she wisely knew was best for me, on the whole.

Was it easy to accept my body in the before photos at the beginning of my journey? Not at first, but then I realised the power of visualisation and keeping my end goal at the forefront of my mind as a way to embody the leaner, fitter, vibrant version of myself. Then it became easier.

As we've discussed earlier, according to Dr Joe Dispenza, when we transform our negativity internally, your body doesn't know if it's real or not and will act as if it is.

Another way to really transform the negative self-talk about your current body is to show gratitude for all that your body can do. There will always be someone in a less fortunate position who would be willing in a heartbeat to exchange places with you, so focusing on all that your body can do for you and has done for you, will help to erase any unfavourable self-talk.

You'll find by doing this, you'll start to see your body with beautiful rose-coloured glasses, and by accepting your body as it is right now, in its beautiful form, you'll be amazed how much easier it will be for you to start losing the weight.

Sounds backwards right?

Another tactic according to the *Law of Attraction* is to have unwavering faith in your body for all it can do but to detach from any outcome so that you already love the body you are in, right now.

Detachment requires you not to obsess over your desired outcome all while having unwavering faith that your desire will come true, as and when it's supposed to. Of course, you need to do the work to head in the right direction, but as I outline in this book, it's small changes over the long-term that will heed the most significant results.

Growing old gracefully.

Another biggie for me and most likely for you.

Discovering more grey hairs or changes in your body or hormones, a couple of extra laugh lines appear. It's pretty confronting, right?

If that's not enough to remind you of your mortality then ageing parents, friends and relatives passing away, children growing up and friends (or even yourself) becoming grandparents; it's the icing on the cake.

We are here for a good time, not a long time as my father has always liked to say, so accepting the ageing process, but appreciating you have the power to slow this down somewhat is very important in my very own philosophy to transform my own body.

**Accept what I can't change and change what I can.
Growing older is inevitable, ageing is a choice.**

Your desire to change versus your acceptance of self

Does one need to be more than the other? Accepting yourself where you are right now, versus it being a reminder of how you got here versus wanting a different future.

Accepting your situation right now and being ok with it means you're less likely to make any significant lifestyle change. And that's ok. But if you're reading this book, I'm assuming you do want to make some improvements to your health, well-being and weight, and therefore your desire to make these changes must be higher than your level of acceptance with where you are right now. This doesn't mean that you can only have one without the other, however.

Jim Fortin, a high-performance leader who uses brain-based behavioural science to mentor some of the world's highest performing people in business, politics and global affairs, shares this about using a higher sense of awareness to solve your problems:

Einstein said, "A problem can never be solved at the level it was created."

Meaning – if you used your current level of thinking to create a problem how do you expect to use that same level of thinking to resolve the issue? Exactly why many people stay stuck in their heads for years or a lifetime.

Ironically, it's not thinking that gives you all the answers you need in life, it's working from higher sense and awareness. Higher mind.

So, with this in mind, your current state of self-acceptance is necessary, but your motivation to evolve to your desired body and mind needs to take the front seat.

Keep quiet – initially

This transformation you're about to embark on is a highly personal experience. My recommendation is that you keep the initial phase to yourself until you've had some time to bed down your new habits and behaviours.

Well-meaning friends can unwittingly sabotage your efforts in the beginning and derail your resolve to improve your health and well-being.

"Oh, come on, one little drink/bite/piece can't hurt".

Even when your friends and loved ones are well aware of your desire to improve your lifestyle, perhaps you've even been established with your transformation for a few months, it can still be unhelpful.

"You've changed", is one I heard from a friend of mine when I politely declined the usual end of week wine at the Rugby club, opting for a glass of water instead.

My answer at the time was "actually I haven't that much, I've returned to how I used to be back in the day pre-children..." but that wasn't entirely true when I think back to the exchange.

What I really should have said was "Thank goodness!" Because in truth, change and growth are inevitable aren't they? As *Eat Pray Love* author Elizabeth Gilbert wrote about in a Face-book post labelled *Beware of Tribal Shame*, when one of us begin to shift away from the pack, it can present social challenges amongst your usual group.

Don't be disheartened, however. Remain strong to your own

convictions, while remaining polite and non-defensive. In time
you may just see some subtle changes in your own peer group,
as I have over the last few months, and you never know, maybe
you had a part to play in that.

I didn't tell anyone what I was doing except my husband. I
didn't even tell my best friends until I had a handle on my slowly
evolving new lifestyle, but also then I would only tell them if the
opportunity arose.

Being off social media also helped me to focus on what I was
doing without letting the cat out of the bag prematurely. I'll
share more about that in *Chapter 2: Creating the Space & Clearing
the Chaos.*

Imagine your very own reveal to your personal friends,
family and the world when you have your dream body.

Core values

Have you ever taken the time to outline or understand what
your very own core values are?

What are core values?

Core value *noun*

Plural noun: **core values**

I. A principle or belief that a person or organisation views as
being of central importance. "*The editor wants to attract more
young readers to the paper while maintaining its core values.*"

Chances are you've worked for a company that has them
outlined along with their mission and vision statements somewhere prominent so staff and customers can see them.

But is it vital for you to have them too?

For sure! Core values will help guide your behaviour and life
choices. Taking the time to delve deep into what your own core
values are will give you clarity and purpose in most aspects of
your life.

Decisions will become effortless, and your personal sense of fulfilment will be the norm when you have guiding principles with which to live your life.

Many of us wander through our life without actually defining or prioritising our guiding life principles or practices to move closer to your fullest potential. According to Abraham Maslow, the American psychologist who created *Maslow's Hierarchy of Needs*, this is called "self-actualisation" and is the pinnacle of existence.

Basic Human Needs

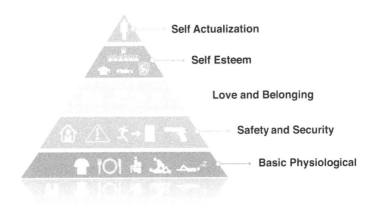

Understanding and outlining your core values will add meaning and direction to your life and be crucial to the ongoing success of your body transformation.

Have a think about what you feel should be the guiding principles of your own life, and how they align with your needs. For example, if one of your values is trust, there's a fair chance you need to be surrounded by people you trust to feel safe. If trust is one of your highest values, this might be why you've never gelled with previous personal trainers – because you haven't sensed a compatible connection with them. There is no right or wrong answer as your very own may be vastly different or similar to mine, based on your own upbringing, culture, traditions and other priorities. This is your life, so it's your choice.

Do consider not overwhelming yourself with too many values which will cause confusion or ambiguity. Limit your list to help keep you on track.

Reflect on values that will take you from where you are now to the person you wish to be, and how you want to live. What will add quality to your years, your own development, and happiness?

Think back to times in your life when you have felt your best or been at your peak. What were you doing or being in these moments in your life? What have been some of your most significant achievements and successes? When has life felt like you were in flow with it and everything felt so right, life couldn't get any better? Pay attention to the details surrounding this time in your life to help craft your own core value set.

It could be when you were a child and were selected to represent your school in a sport, or you won the award for art. Perhaps it was when you decided to try *Dry January*, and it lasted a whole three months, and you saved money and some hangovers. Maybe it was that time you decided to save money for your overseas holiday, so you set a budget and stuck to it, to have the holiday of a lifetime. Perhaps you were offered your dream job or given a promotion. Or it was the time you bought your first property.

Likewise, think back to some of your not so great moments in life and remember where you were. What decision led you there or away from there? Perhaps it was the type of relationship you were in or the overindulgent behaviour you were engaging in. Maybe you're not being present with your children or partner. Perhaps you're feeling neglected in your relationship, but possibly you're being neglectful too. Or you're neglecting your own needs. Maybe this is you now, and you know you're not making the ideal daily decisions or behaviours to feel your best. Take note of what's happening around you right now, and how you'd like to improve on this.

What are your needs and how do they connect to your core values?

You may decide yours are:

- putting your family and relationship first,
- a career or business you love or feel valued in,
- quality and enjoyable life-sustaining food,
- focus on enjoyable fitness & movement, and
- quality time spent with like-minded friends having fun and top quality.

Focus on the feeling

When we are making any significant changes to the way we currently operate, it can sometimes seem like life wants to conspire against us, or we put up some form of resistance. It's all too hard we might tell ourselves, as we fall back into old patterns.

Rather than focus on how complicated the changes are, why not focus on how you want to feel. Rather than being preoccupied on the outcome, start becoming mindful of the inner self-talk you are having, and try to rewire your mind, to attach a positive feeling to the work you are going to be doing on not only bettering your health but creating a brand-new version of you.

Rather than dreading the gym, why not focus on how you are going to feel following your workout and how much stronger you will be.

Rather than the self-talk that you aren't a good cook, ask yourself how you will feel by taking charge of your health by knowing precisely what premium fuel you are giving it to perform.

Rather than thinking that every meal should be a celebration, re-train yourself to know that food is for fuel and energy and that feasting like in the middle ages is for special occasions not breakfast, lunch and dinner.

Rather than rewarding yourself with a treat meal, think of non-food related treats you can pay yourself, like some park time with your kids, going for a morning walk with a girlfriend, getting your nails done, receiving a massage or wrapping yourself up with a blanket and a good romance novel. Or binge-watching a couple of your favourites on *Netflix*. Whatever you enjoy that isn't food related.

The waiting room

After a few months of embracing this new lifestyle, my husband was inspired to give his own body transformation a try.

One weekend during the beginning of his own journey, having made some adjustments to our usually full and active social life, he jokingly asked me "so what are we supposed to do while we wait for our hot bodies?"

We laughed and called this time *"The Waiting Room"*.

But rather than focus on the things we were missing out on, I encouraged us to look at the things we were opening ourselves up to. We had more energy, and time to spend with our children, more time to develop other interests and hobbies that were often put in the 'when we have more time' pile, more family outdoor activity time, and a general feeling of cleaning up other areas of our lives that would sometimes feel chaotic. Plus, the lure of better health and longevity was very appealing and sexy, especially having each other to encourage along this path.

Robyn's recommendations

Claim your own core values by writing them down in your journal or somewhere prominent for you to see often. But don't just write them down. Act on them. Use them to help make your decisions and guide your choices.

They may be subject to change as you test them against different scenarios, and you home in on honestly what kind of life and person you wish to be at your highest version.

THE BODY PLAN (ON ONE PAGE)

What does The Body Plan look like? Here's a picture for you! And a quick overview of the 6 stages.

THE BODY PLAN

STEP 1
Setting Your
Intentions

STEP 2
Creating the Space &
Clearing the Chaos

STEP 3
Keeping Records

STEP 4
Understanding
Flexible Dieting

STEP 5
Planning Ahead

STEP 6
Sustaining Your
Progress

PART II

FOUNDATION KNOWLEDGE: PRE-PREP STAGE

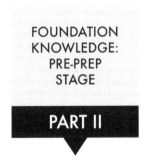

So why is the preparation stage so important? Without mentally preparing yourself and having all the tools and resources necessary to give your transformation a red-hot go, you'll be operating in more of a reactive response than proactive.

It's more than likely that the tools and advice I suggest in *The Body Plan* are a departure from your standard operating system, which means there is a higher risk for stress and anxiety as you learn new skills and develop your new and improved mindset.

To be prepared will help to reduce the need to be in constant react mode and enable you to devote your time to where it's needed most, and that is in acquiring your new skills and habits.

What I realised with all my past failed attempts at maintaining a healthy body fitness and weight level, was that I'd dive right in without the proper preparation and end up failing at the first sign of a challenge.

I believe the key to long-lasting success is a solid preparation phase and that there are three fairly distinct stages – missing any of which will end up spelling disaster for your weight loss and health goals. They are:

1. Setting your intentions,
2. Creating the space and clearing the chaos, and
3. Keeping records.

So, let's dive in, with *Chapter 1: Setting Your Intentions*.

CHAPTER 1: SETTING YOUR INTENTIONS

*W*hen you don't set your intentions, you don't end up having a clear end goal and when you don't have a definite end goal what happens? In short, you have nothing to direct your energy towards, so your attempt has failed before it even begins. No one wants that, do they? But it's the main reason why so many efforts fail, and it's really not that hard to get your head around properly before you start.

What does setting your intentions involve precisely?

- knowing when you're going to start,
- reflecting on your past,
- knowing what got you to where you're at now,
- defining what you want your 'future' self to look and feel like,
- getting honest with yourself, and
- setting your goals.

So, let's get started with that first step for setting clear intentions – knowing when you're going to start.

Set the date

Make the commitment.

Enough is enough.

You've hit rock bottom.

You've been talking about doing this for months, maybe years.

Select a day to get mentally prepared to dedicate your full attention to this.

Be intentional.

Prioritise yourself, so that your loved ones will reap the benefits as will you.

It's time to roll up your sleeves and get serious.

Choose a day that will be the most practical for you for your weekly ongoing check-in day. I like Sunday as it's the beginning of our work week where we live in the Middle East. You may wish to elect a Monday or even a Friday before your weekend begins; it's entirely personal and entirely up to you.

It may be tomorrow, or it may be two weeks from now, it may be after you finish moving to a new house next month or when you get back from holidays, but don't delay too long or else that day will never come. Just be realistic and know that your time is here.

Keep in mind that you'll need to allow time to acquire the equipment that I talked about in *How to Use This Book*.

You can download your own checklist here in your free starter kit http://bit.ly/bodyplanstarter

Whether you make it as easy as going to your local store to buy or purchasing online, this prior preparation will form part of your success.

Robyn's recommendation

Select a start date that is the most practical for you to sustain for ongoing check-ins. You will continue to use this day of the week to record your weekly progress, keeping in mind your weekly schedule is the best idea for ongoing success.

Write this start date in your diary, on your mirror, on your fridge, in your electronic calendar, everywhere you can see it. And remember, as I said in *Part I*, keep the visualisation of your final result in your mind.

"The reason most people never reach their goals is that they don't define them, or even seriously consider them as believable or achievable."
    Denis Watley

The past you

When it comes down to it, without having a goal to strive towards, you're really floating along aimlessly without much hope of hitting any kind of target.

But before we focus on getting what you want your future to look like, I'd like to invite you to do some reflecting first.

Despite living by the rule of having no regrets and not looking backwards, I do think it is essential that you take stock and give gratitude for where the past has brought you. To assess the behaviours and habits and how they may have impacted your journey to this current point. This will help you have a better understanding of how to modify yourself and take actions based here in the present, so you can start the journey to your future.

I mean it when I say your journey first begins within. It's all good and well to say you want to lose ten kilos this year, or start prioritising your own self-care, however, if you don't have a greater understanding of who you are and how you tick, you may be challenged when it comes to making the transition to a different way of living.

This might hurt, but the way you've been previously operating isn't working. So, before we can even look at setting some goals as it will be helpful to truly understand what needs to change, then plot how to get there from here.

Real and lasting change comes from within first.

Take responsibility and acknowledge your previous choices, circumstances and actions that have led you to here. Then make a declaration to your health and happiness, that you are ready to make the 'uncomfortable at times, but highly rewarding' modifications from here on in.

If you've struggled with your weight for some time, it's not your fault. You don't lack discipline, willpower or the desire to get in shape. So please stop beating yourself up!

Our body is perfect but she's in charge, and even though we can try to trick her by trying the latest fad diet in the short-term, she will win out in the end.

Her main job is to keep us safe and alive, and even though we no longer need to be lean to run from predators or gain body fat to protect our organs for the harsh winter, our incredible machines are still made of the same components they used to be, before industrialisation.

Our body controls our appetite, metabolism, cravings and energy levels. To keep us alive or safe, she will switch on specific chemicals to ensure she does her job.

She doesn't want to punish us; her main focus is survival.

When she doesn't feel safe, she will do whatever it takes, and for that, we should honour her.

Mental and emotional stress is understood in much the same way by our body as a physical threat – and will react as if she is being ambushed, by chemically orchestrating what she was designed to do. Protect you.

Even ongoing daily grind stress can compound over time to have a similar result.

Addressing your stress and emotional triggers first and foremost should be your priority if you're serious about getting healthier and losing your excess flab.

Guess what? Dieting is a form of stress too, and when you don't first address the internal triggers for your weight gain, you will continue to yo-yo, with the starvation/binge cycles leaving you frustrated and often more overweight than before.

So, you see losing weight isn't just about energy in, energy out. It's definitely a component of a weight loss plan, but I couldn't even dream about having long-term and enjoyable weight loss if I failed to do the work on my emotional and mental health.

Over to you:

- Why do you feel your current diet is flawed?
- Can you pinpoint a specific incident when your weight began to increase?
- What's your body trying to tell you?
- What are you most proud of from the past year?
- What were your biggest challenges from the previous year?
- What have you learnt about yourself this past year?
- What can you now release?
- What made you happy this past year?
- What can you do to focus first on healing your *Mind*

and *Soul* before you even start to see the work show
up on your beautiful *Body*?

- What are you most thankful for from this past year?
- What more can you say to complete your year from
  now? (Include good, bad and indifferent.)

Robyn's recommendation

If you can pinpoint an exact moment or incident or trauma
when your weight began to increase, or a series of events, I urge
you to deal with this in the best way you can via therapy or
professional support. Working through this pain and discomfort
may be a challenge, but it's often the very cause and reason for
you to remain where you're at.

With the above reflective questions, it's time to now forgive,
release, and let go. Thank your previous self for all the learnings,
growth and support and say:

**"Thank you for showing me to learn from my past. Thank you
for the value of my previous lessons, and now I shall."**

The present you

Now that you've taken a good look down memory lane and
realised the pleasing aspects of your past you want to carry
forward and the challenges and aspects of you and your history
that you are now ready to release, let's look at you now.

"How did I get here?" You might be asking yourself.

Were you previously naturally slim and did not need to
watch what you ate? Or maybe you've always been carrying a
little bit of extra padding, but it's gradually increased over time
to a point you don't recognise yourself anymore. Or maybe
you've always been in a yo-yo diet cycle.

"Who is this person?" you may ask.

In regard to my own journey, before I could get clear on where I wanted to go *(future)*, I needed to take stock of where I was at right now *(present)*.

Take some time to reflect and answer the following questions honestly and thoughtfully before moving to your present day, re-visiting what your core values are and how you wish to show up in the world in line with them.

Let's take a look at you, at this moment – right now.

- Why do you want this body transformation?
- How are you feeling right now?
- What are you most looking forward to?
- Is there anything you are least looking forward to?
- What changes are you hoping to see in 1 month?
- What changes are you hoping to see in 3 months?
- What changes are you hoping to see in 6 months?
- What changes are you hoping to see in 12 months?
- What changes are you wishing to experience beyond the next year or two?
- What are you going to do, to help yourself move forward towards your goal/s?
- Who are you going to be, to help yourself move forward towards your goal/s?

Future you

_____

Success leaves clues, and if you sow the same seeds, you'll reap the same rewards.
   Brad Thor

_____

Time to fast forward to the future you and set some goals of precisely what you desire for your whole self. *Mind, Body* and *Soul*.

Sit for a moment and really think about where you want to be in twelve months. Visualise your ideal day, how it looks and feels to you.

Dr Joe Dispenza in his book *Breaking the Habit of Being Yourself: How to Lose Your Mind and Create a New One*, talks about how you can improve your life and habits, by first changing your personality. It all begins with a *thought*, then a *feeling* then, *being*. Here we are going to home in on the thinking and feeling before we work on the being.

It might sound severe to want or need to change your personality, but if you genuinely want to change the way you show up in this very short life we've been gifted, visiting the root of who you are and why you do things will help you to pivot and improve so you can ultimately be the best you.

It's never too late, don't give up on yourself. You owe it to you. Just like I owed it to myself.

The ULTIMATE Version of You

This could be realistic or nonsensical according to you, but the idea is to really home in on what your ultimate desired outcome or vision of you will look like, starting from the smallest little details.

- What time of day will you get up?
- How will you feel upon waking?
- Where will you be living?
- What will you do as soon as you wake up?
- What clothes will you be wearing?

- What will you eat for breakfast and where will you be eating it and who will you be with?
- What will you do after breakfast?
- Who will you be spending time with today?
- What will you eat for lunch and where will you eat it and who will you be with?
- How will you spend your time in the afternoon?
- What will you eat for dinner and where will you eat it and who will you be with?
- How will you spend your time after dinner?
- What time will you go to bed?
- How do you want to feel?

For example, I kept a future perception of me with:

- A lean, pain-free body, with slight muscle definition not unlike a bikini or fitness model,
- Feminine but strong,
- Wearing fitted clothes bought off the rack, not my usual floaty, shapeless, baggy kaftans,
- Only one chin,
- Well rested,
- Chilled out, and
- Exuding patience with my loved ones, well really with everyone to be honest.

I also visualised revealing myself to my family and friends in Australia who hadn't seen me for a year, wowing them at my new me. And you know what? This actually happened. On our last visit home, my father, a veteran personal trainer, pulled me aside and said he was really pleased to see I had made such a positive lifestyle change which not only impacted how I looked, but he noticed how much more energy I had as well as a vast improvement in disposition.

Part of the visualisation process I did was to have a calm and trusting confidence that at some point soon, people would be seeing my new body and asking how the hell I did it.

Robyn's recommendation

Now visualise precisely how you will look and feel in twelve months. This is your ideal vision of you.

Describe, draw, create a vision board or a *Pinterest* board (you can make it private if you wish) on how you want to look and feel – do not hold back! The clearer you get on this vision, the closer you will get to making it a reality because everything that you do and achieve always began as a thought first.

Part of my own process wasn't just to focus on the outcome but also the feeling that the result would derive for me. Taking steps to embody that feeling before hitting my goal would bring it much closer. This will keep you grounded, focused and motivated. Not just the number on the scale.

I highly recommend Danielle La Porte and her book *The Desire Map: A Guide to Creating Goals with Soul* if you wish to explore goal setting further and life-planning tactics that are rooted in your core desired feelings. She explains an approach to goal setting, so you are no longer chasing the goal but the emotion you want from achieving said goal.

I promise you, if I can accomplish this body transformation, you can too.

Your results are going to vary due to the uniqueness of you; however, the more honest you are with yourself, the easier it will be to move closer towards your goal. 400-500g/1lb weight loss per week is an average I have sustained. In my experience, any more than that can be too rapid for sustainability over the long-term. Any less means you might need to tweak your intake to help you move through the ups and downs of fat loss because it is not linear at all. For anyone.

It's time to imagine who you want to be in the future and embody everything about her, spirit and mind as though that day is now; it's already happened.

1. Know clearly and precisely the type of body you desire. Is she muscular and athletic, or lean and thin? See in your mind's eye exactly how you want to look and feel.

2. Envisage yourself looking like this right now, having already achieved it, as though it's actual. How do you feel?

3. Assume the role of that desired version of yourself. Experience it as a foregone conclusion, no excuse. You embody this version of you now. That's who you are. Right here, right now. Trust that as you visualise yourself in this way, you are bringing it closer to reality.

4. Embody it. Feel it. Speak it. It's the truth. Use the present tense as if it's here now.

Get real

I had to get brutally honest with myself about my weight and how much I needed to lose so that I could have a real-life target to hit.

It's confronting to be extremely honest with yourself by claiming your starting point, but to experience the sweetness of your success, no matter how painful it feels in the beginning, will require you to have a baseline. If you ignore this crucial step, it won't feel nearly so good when you start to experience your progress.

How can you manage something you can't measure?

To begin, I calculated my current and then ideal (goal) weight range (notice I said range and not actual weight) by checking my *BMI.* You can find online calculators all over the internet, or check out my own here http://bit.ly/bodyplancalc

Many will argue that the *BMI* formula is not a hundred per cent accurate and may not take into account things like body type, but like much of what I will share with you in this book, in my experience this is just as much an art as it is a science. Using some or all of these tools will help to give you a ballpark figure to generate your own unique starting point. Then we can begin to put the puzzle pieces together for your own unique picture.

Robyn's recommendation

Calculate your current *BMI* and write it down, then determine what range you'd like to aim towards for our goal setting which is yet to come. Alternatively, you may have a previous ideal weight range that you'd want to return to. If it's realistic, then aim for it.

Goal setting: good, better, best

Even though I don't agree with setting yourself a strict timeline for when to hit your ultimate target, I do think it's important to have a desired and defined best case scenario outcome.

If you don't set your destination, then how will you be able to map out and head in the correct direction?

It may take months or even years to hit your ideal goal if you wish to do it the same way I have, with pleasure and sustainability. I am yet to achieve mine at the time of publishing, but I am getting closer each day using the principles and methods I outline in this book. I do believe; however, it's crucial to have mini-milestones (kedges as discussed in *Part I: Mind*) along the way to fuel your sense of achievement and keep your motivation high.

So, here's what my ultimate goals looked like:

- Weight goal =
- Body fat per cent goal =
- Dress/jean size =
- Reduction or elimination of back pain & hip pain,
- Reduction in cholesterol, and
- Reduction in blood sugar and diabetes risk reduced or eliminated.

So far, I have already achieved a reduction of back and hip pain, cholesterol and blood sugar levels and I have almost hit my overall weight loss goal.

Examples of some mini-milestones that I have set for myself over the entire duration of my *Body Transformation* have been:

- five to seven kilo weight loss,
- learning and perfecting three new family-friendly recipes for dinner and lunch prep per month,
- twice a week at Pilates to help strengthen my core,
- twice a week heavy weight lifting, and
- reverse dieting when I hit a consistent plateau (not something I will cover in this book as it's not a focus for the first three months).

Ideally, your mini-milestones should be one thing that you

can achieve in three months. Because in this book I'm only focusing on what you need to know for the first three-month period, I would suggest a mini-milestone would be something like a two to three kilo weight loss and success with creating an achievable new nutritional diet practice.

If you prefer a more relaxed but less precise approach to goal setting, focusing on improving one or two things each week or month is a great goal to have, depending on your current life responsibilities, but don't use that as a crutch either. You can and will make the time for those things that are important to you. In the very least, aim to be better at something this week that you weren't doing so well last week. This will become clearer as you work through this book.

Robyn's recommendation

Write down your aesthetic and non-aesthetic goals and keep them somewhere visible that you will see every day. On your bathroom mirror, on the fridge, in the car, on your phone screensaver. Consider breaking them down into short-term and long-term but also be open to them taking a longer or shorter time as I've previously discussed with eliminating timelines.

CHAPTER 2: CREATING THE SPACE AND CLEARING THE CHAOS

*N*ow that you've set your outcome goals, you really need to plot out 'the how' which will form part of the process.

Where most fail is in the implementation and carving out space in their diary to achieve what they desire.

They might set a goal to hit the gym three times a week, but don't physically look at their schedule to commit to when they will do it or how they can practically fit it in.

Others say they don't have time to be healthy, but they spend more time than they can afford scrolling through *Facebook* or watching mindless television before they go to bed each night.

In this next chapter, I'm going to share with you tips and places where I was able to recover more time and space to open up for the healthful pursuits I'd been wanting to follow.

To give yourself this gift for the next three months and set yourself up for the rest of your life, you will need to find extra space and make sacrifices to other time that drains your life right now, and is not getting you where you really desire to be.

How can you create the luxury of space and reduce the chaos in your every day?

I'll talk about:

- managing stress,
- social media control,
- optimal sleep practices,
- regulating your environment,
- recognising why multi-tasking isn't ideal, and
- learning how to say no.

Let's dive into the big one, *managing your stress*.

Managing stress

Many of us waste unnecessary time dealing with the after-effects of harmful stress in our life.

In some instances, good stress is healthy for us and can get us moving in the intended direction of our dreams, but if you're often feeling:

- maxed out,
- tired,
- angry,
- low motivation,
- aches and pains, and
- low energy

then chances are you need to re-evaluate life and how you currently live it before it gets the better of you.

Years ago, in London, while at dinner, I sat next to a freelance fashion photographer. He shared with me a story about an elderly

Buddhist monk he had befriended at Heathrow airport while they both waited to board a flight to New York. Curious to learn why a Buddhist monk was going to such an urban place like Manhattan, he struck up a conversation. The monk said he'd been invited to participate in a research project on his experience with longevity due to his alarmingly good health at such a ripe old age.

The photographer asked the monk why he thought he had lived so long and so healthfully.

The monk believed it was due to a life lived free or low in stress. His life philosophy was that nothing was off limits, but anything to excess or intoxication was not ideal. Therefore, if he enjoyed one cigarette and the act of having only one reduced his stress levels, then it was beneficial to his overall health and well-being.

The photographer offered to take some headshots of the monk in Central Park as a gift, and when the photographs were ready for delivery, he tried to contact the monk to make necessary arrangements. Sadly, the monk had passed away according to his travel companion. The companion speculated the monk had died due to the environmental stress he'd been under while staying in bustling and chaotic New York City, a vastly different environment to his monastery at home.

Here are some ways that I have found to help manage my own stress levels:

- creating more white space in my otherwise full schedule,
- managing my environment,
- prioritising sleep,
- reduction or elimination of multi-tasking,
- being more active,
- increasing fun,

- reducing or eliminating perfectionistic tendencies, and
- being of service to others (especially those in need).

Finding and applying supportive tools to help with stress management can assist with your own success and life satisfaction. I personally developed my personal *stress toolkit*, to assist with managing my own stress levels.

My stress management toolkit

1. **Exercise:** In the first three months, I don't use training as a weight loss tool at all. I imagine my exercise as a pill I take to regulate my stress, emotional and mental state. I always feel so good for the rest of the day following a good intense workout or an in-depth Pilates session. Even after a long brisk walk around my neighbourhood. Just to clarify again this wasn't a focus for the first three months of my body transformation as a weight loss tool.

2. **Reading:** I have always loved to read (and write), and over the years I've found less time available to do so. Now I allocate time in my schedule to enjoy a good fiction book to escape, where I can, and the results on my stress levels speak for themselves.

3. **Essential oils:** topically and diffusing them in the house and car, you can find an essential oil to support you, from gifting you extra energy to aiding your immune system. Introducing essential oils and aromatherapy to our family has been one of the best things we've done in the last couple of years to manage behaviour and mood as well as overall

health. Even my seven-year-old's teacher noticed a positive difference in his focus and attitude at school since we started using essential oils.

4. **Meditation:** this is not a strong point of mine, but something I try to do when I can but not in the traditional sense. I consider my long walks without any distraction like earphones as my meditation or even a long hot bath by candlelight.

5. **Journaling:** there is no right or wrong way to journal, however many have claimed its' powers in helping to deepen your connection with yourself. It involves a practice of writing, drawing, or creating in a practice that has no rules. If you'd like to learn more about this, I highly recommend Julia Cameron's *The Artist's Way,* where she dives deep into a practice known as *Morning Pages.*

Robyn's recommendation

Come up with your own version of a *stress management toolkit.*

As adults, many of us have lost what lights us up and are clueless about our favourite interests and pastimes. Spend some quiet time reflecting on hobbies that you once enjoyed that you haven't made time to enjoy these days.

One of mine mentioned above is reading. I used to devour books and still have a vast collection that doesn't get as much attention these days.

Mediation, dancing, massage, masturbation or lovemaking with your partner or anything that you know just makes you feel good that you've been denying yourself can all form part of your very own stress relief toolkit.

I have recently taken up singing and drum lessons, which is something that I've always wanted to do. Not only has it been filling my soul on an entirely new level but is also an excellent way to bond with my seven-year-old, who is also learning the drums. Having something in common that we both share is priceless and fulfilling for not just me but him too.

I have found in my experience being disconnected from self and what makes you happy is often the most significant cause of general dissatisfaction and subsequent weight gain.

Get to know yourself again which is often hard for us mothers who live for everyone else except ourselves for a period in our lives. It is not selfish to give back to yourself, just like the airline oxygen analogy.

Your *stress toolkit* may look similar or very different to mine but getting to know yourself again will be imperative to managing your stress.

You'll be a better mother, wife, friend, daughter and outright person when your own cup is not depleted, and you are able to give back to your loved ones.

Social media

Earlier I spoke about getting off social media.

Several tech executives have recently spoken up over their concerns about social media and the effect it is having on our society.

Chamath Palihapitiya, a former *Facebook* executive, said in December 2017 that he has "tremendous guilt" about the company he helped make. *"I think we have created tools that are ripping apart the social fabric of how society works,"* according to an article in the Washington Post. I tend to agree.

As someone who has spent a great deal of the last 15 years as a heavy technology user, from sharing my overseas life and travels with family using a now-defunct *Myspace* account to be an early adopter with *Facebook* and then other blogging platforms, I'm no stranger to the positives of the *World Wide Web*. Not to mention my pre-teen education in programming computers.

Despite this, I made a decision in 2016 to take a break from using my social media accounts to focus on the life that was in front of me, in the real world.

Initially, I was inspired by Kelsey Byers in her *Eat Clean and Follow Your Dreams* eBook, a fitness model who lost forty pounds and became a fitness blogger. I resonated with her philosophy *"there is always someone getting a workout in while you are surfing the internet."*

I completely deactivated my *Facebook* profile and only kept *Facebook Messenger* on my *iPhone* for keeping in touch with family and friends. As an expat living abroad this kind of connection was still vital for me to remain close to loved ones but not the other 1600 people, I am 'friends' with.

Getting off social media this way might seem severe, but personally, I needed to remove the distractions that were keeping me from my goals. I also needed to break the habit of checking in with what the rest of the world was doing. By doing this, it gave me the equivalent of enough hours to open me up to reading sometimes two to three books a week. Imagine that!

Don't get me wrong, previously I've suggested ways to reduce stress in your life, and I understand many people use social media and the internet after a full day of work to decompress and relax. However, for most people, the use of social media can have the opposite effect of what you began to use it for.

How many times have you found yourself hopping on your phone or laptop to just check-in with what your friends are doing online and two hours later you're still online mindlessly watching funny videos and looking at friend's photos of their last weekend's barbecue? Or perhaps comparing your life to the highlight reel of a long-lost high school friend?

No, you don't? Well, your self-control and awareness are way better than mine.

Kind of embarrassing really, that I found myself grabbing my phone first thing in the morning, before jumping out of bed, to check my *Facebook, Instagram, What's App* and email before even saying good morning to my kids.

And although there is plenty to be grateful for with technology these days, there is also a dark side to it that is hard to shake if you're not being mindful of your internet usage.

The Center for Humane Technology says that social media has *"trained us to replace our self-worth with likes, encourages comparison with others, and creates the constant illusion of missing out."*

So, I went completely cold turkey, off all social media for a minimum of six months. And that is saying a lot for someone like me that relied heavily on social media for the running and marketing of my work, plus staying connected to family overseas.

Want to know what happened? Well besides my weight loss? I became more present with my kids, I had way more time for myself, I stopped comparing myself to strangers and even other friends on the internet, my relationship with my husband strengthened, I read an average of four books a month (that's four more a month than I was reading before) and I felt less anxiety in general.

I focused on more in-person connections, and I was able to detox myself of the need to always be checking in with friends and people I follow online.

Did I return to social media?

Yes, I did, but I was able to look at it for the tool it is, and manage my usage of it a lot better, with greater awareness, self-control and intuition.

I still need to be extremely mindful of spending too much

time on the interwebs, but these days I am more conscious of when I've been adding value or wasting time in my life.

Robyn's recommendation

Think of all the times you've spent on social media or your smartphone this week. What could you have done with your time instead?

As Alexandra Franzen says in her blog post titled *"Why I don't use social media anymore"*;

"At the end of my life, will I say to myself: 'My God, I am so grateful that I tweeted 151,200 times (2,016 tweets per year times seventy-five years starting around age twenty-five) throughout my life? Time well spent! How wonderful! Alex, is this really how you want to be spending your life-minutes? Isn't there something else that might be a more meaningful use of your time? Wouldn't you rather be walking outside, talking to your mom, writing a novel, having sex, working out, mailing a letter, volunteering, you know, all of those things that you 'never have enough time' to do?'"

How is social media helping and how is it hurting your life?

Allocate time for your personal goals first in your schedule before allowing yourself to sit down to get on the internet.

Sleep

Unhealthy sleep habits were my modus operandi, before my body transformation. While running my business and having had two children just short of two years apart, as most parents will attest to, good quality sleep doesn't get much attention especially during those early years of parenthood.

Then bad habits continued and, in a bid, to have child-free time in the evening, staying up later than I should was the norm.

In my previous pre 'body transformation life', I would more

often than not, crawl into bed after eleven pm. Usually, I'd be fighting sleep by seven pm, but after winding myself up with computer, television or a bottle of wine (sometimes all three), I'd find it hard to calm my mind and not get to bed until late. Self-medicating with the wine no doubt added to my poor-quality sleep.

I'd then struggle to get out of bed in the morning, always assuming I just wasn't naturally a morning person. I've forever been known in my family for loving my sleep, and despite always wanting to be a 'fresh out of bed in the morning' person, I just could never manage it. Even at high school and university, I'd be pulling in my best assignments at one am in the morning before the due date.

But this all changed with my body transformation. Once I made the call to get off social media and became more strategic with my fitness, I found bed beckoning me shortly after putting my kids to bed between seven and eight o'clock in the evening.

Of course, it helped that my husband also had an extremely early start in the morning and would be tucked up in bed by eight-thirty pm. Before long I was falling into bed before nine pm myself and waking up so much fresher in the mornings.

Most people require at least seven hours of sleep to feel human. I'm being honest here, I really do need about eight hours minimum to feel normal and not hit the mid-afternoon slump.

It might seem like a sacrifice to your already premium free time in the evening, but for the benefit of more energy and better moods through the day, I am happy to crawl into bed much earlier these days to bounce out of bed in the mornings, ready to take on whatever the day has to give me.

At times I do feel like the weekdays do fly by in a haze of school runs, making lunches, dinner prep, kids' activities and errand running. But in the end, it makes me appreciate the downtime on the weekends that much more. On the plus side, more and better-quality sleep helps with stress management and might seem counterproductive to creating more space in your day, but better sleep definitely creates more quality in my day.

Now my evenings are heavily protected, and very little will get me out of the house in the evening these days. I value my rest and how much it has improved the quality of my life.

Why is sleep so critical to weight loss?

There are two hunger hormones called ghrelin and leptin. In short, ghrelin signals hunger when your stomach is empty, and it's getting close to meal time, and leptin suppresses hunger and messages to your brain feelings of fullness.

When you have less than optimum sleep, your body produces more ghrelin and a lower amount of leptin, which makes you feel hungrier and increases your appetite.

When you get inadequate sleep, your body also produces more of the stress hormone cortisol which is linked to weight gain and increased hunger.

As an ex-flight attendant who used to work in many time zones and live in a constant state of jet lag and shift work haze, I can testify to when you're tired but required to remain awake and alert, eating more for an increase in energy. I do have such fond memories of raiding the delicious desserts and gourmet sandwiches from *First* and *Business* class cabins after the primary food and beverage service were complete and the passengers were all taken care of.

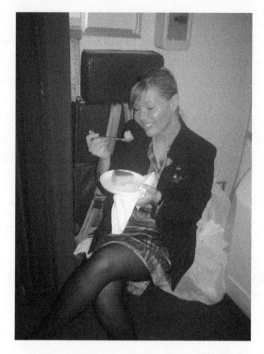

On meal break, Business Class cabin, QANTAS airlines,
2007

One special memory I have from back in my long-haul flying days was during one of our crew scheduled meal breaks. Most of the passengers were sleeping after having been fed, and my favourite cabin manager called those on our break to come up to the *Business* class galley. He had set up a makeshift dining table with linens and all the leftover meals and desserts (crew were typically allowed to eat leftover meals on meal breaks), and we gathered around the 'dining table', to sit on galley metal storage boxes. The only thing missing was some wine, but of course, it's against regulations to drink on the job.

FROM A PRACTICAL POINT OF VIEW, when you have less sleep and more awake time, you've opened up your eating window to be larger, which means more time to be tempted to eat.

Robyn's recommendation

If you know your sleep habits could be improved upon, commit to making small incremental changes over the next couple of weeks, depending on how much extra sleep you need to be dedicated to.

You could try by slowly introducing an extra half an hour each night, or by taking steps to wind down for bed earlier, by enjoying a warm bath, not allowing screens in the bedroom, listening to a calming meditation or some other kind of ritual you can do every night to signify its bedtime.

It may take some getting used to, but rest assured, once you start to implement better sleep practices they will become a healthy habit that you'll begin to protect with all your life.

Managing your environment

Being conscious of where you thrive physically is an essential part of self-awareness.

Over the years, I have gravitated towards a quieter, simpler life, after years of living the jet-set, party-girl lifestyle.

Personally, I now crave the quiet of the suburbs or the ocean, and I don't enjoy being surrounded by too many people at once these days, especially as I now understand myself more as an Empath.

I pick up on other's vibrations whether I know them or not, so even a trip to the local mall during peak time isn't one of my favourite things to do, and I return home feeling drained and depleted.

Many others really thrive in bustling crowds and high-vibe

situations that replenish their energies. Understanding yourself and where you flourish is crucial to helping you make choices that serve your highest-self.

Of course, we cannot always be so controlling of our environment, but getting to know yourself and develop strategies that you can use when it's not ideal will support your mission. Not only is this advantageous for your body transformation but generally in life. Get to know yourself.

Not only is your environment the physical place you put yourself in, but also the people you have around you.

As I mentioned in an earlier chapter, you are the average of the people you surround yourself with. Be conscious of the individuals you spend the most time with. Be intentional and supportive of your needs and goals as much as possible which will fast track your success and general life satisfaction.

In regard to my own body transformation, I found I tend to gravitate towards people who are in better shape, mentally, physically and emotionally, or at least in the trenches with me doing the work on themselves too.

I am able to be inspired by them, work out with them and enjoy being frequently around them, which helps to lift my own vibration. I also hope I have this same impact on them.

That's not to say that all of my friends are fitness models and that I'm superficial by weeding my friends out by the way they look, but it's essential for my own happiness to be around like-minded people who enjoy being active and seek out healthy past-times, whether they look like it or not.

If this is not always possible for you in real life, then you can also seek positive role models online, or in books to keep your own mindset in a positive vibe.

Not everyone in your life is going to be where you want to be, but try to skew it in the direction of where you wish to be.

Robyn's recommendations

Are there any people, situations, environments that you're currently in, that you don't like, feel misaligned or are in opposition to your desired outcome?

Make a list of ways that you can start to add more positive influences in your life or introducing these aspects to your current relationships or situations. For example, rather than seeing your best friend for cocktails, why not meet to walk the dogs or do a gym class then have a smoothie afterwards.

The cost of multi-tasking

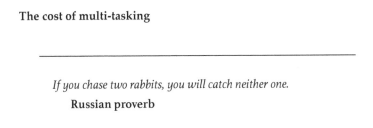

If you chase two rabbits, you will catch neither one.
Russian proverb

Many women claim to be masters of multi-tasking, and wear it like a badge of honour, but is multi-tasking all it's cracked up to be?

A few years back, during a period when I was investing a great deal of my time and money in my business growth and self-development, I came across a theory about multi-tasking. It enlightened me, how performing more than one task at the same time was detrimental to productivity in said tasks.

Gerald M. Weinberg wrote in *Quality Software Management: Systems Thinking* how productivity and quality of work are lost when we attempt to do more than one project at a time.

Although his topic was based on how context switching (multi-tasking) impacts an engineering software team, you can apply his findings to anyone who is trying to do more than one project while simultaneously doing another.

You would experience this loss of attention or productivity yourself when trying to read an email and talking to someone on the telephone. Even though we think we can do both at the same time, we don't give our attention to either 100 per cent.

This is how I approached my body transformation.

While it's not practical for most if not all of us to clear our schedules entirely to focus on only diet and fitness, you can be smart to manage your time as best as your own responsibilities allow.

To apply discernment for the first month of my body transformation I did not focus on any kind of fitness at all until I knew I had my diet, nutrition and meal planning down to an art.

This would enable my new habits to become automatic as I described in the section on *Habit Stacking*.

Of course, I had other focuses in my daily life, like running the household and being the primary caregiver to my children, but I would allocate blocks of time where I could solely focus on meal prep, planning and nutritional education where I could, and not allow any other distractions during those blocks of time, like the washing or *Netflix*.

Robyn's recommendations

Be mindful of being present in each task, whether it's while you're washing the dishes, driving in the car, having a shower or getting on your computer. It's taken me a few years of self-control and mindfulness, but I am less likely to have thirty website tabs open on my laptop these days with now usually a maximum of five. Now I'm more mindful to complete one task before I begin another. And my personal satisfaction is higher because I'm finishing more jobs than ever before.

Learning the art of saying no

You need to learn to be protective of your own personal time if you wish to have success, and in my experience if you make the time for the things that are most important to you, you will achieve your goals. It just depends on how significant this body transformation is to you.

According to the *Four Burner Theory*, to be genuinely successful in one area of your life, you need to be thoughtful about where you dedicate your time.

Each burner represents an aspect of your life: *family, work, health and well-being*, and *social*.

The idea is that to be successful you really need to turn off one burner, but to be hugely successful you'll need to turn off at least two.

In my opinion, it's a personal choice that only you can make, but by using this theory you'll have a higher chance of being a top performer in the chosen parts of your life, rather than being mediocre in all.

It also doesn't need to be forever. Embrace the seasons of life, as the importance of each of these aspects will change. Nothing is permanent, but to achieve your long-lasting goals you will need to adapt your current lifestyle and which burners you have turned up high and those that are switched off, no matter if temporary.

Learning how to say no gracefully to things that are not in line with your higher goals and desires will need to be practised if it's not natural for you, but once you do it a few times it will become easier.

And just like Zdravko Cvijetic says in *Medium*'s most viral article *13 Things You Should Give Up if You Want to Be Successful; "successful people know that in order to accomplish their goals, they will have to say NO to certain tasks, activities, and demands from their friends, family, and colleagues."*

Alexandra Franzen, in her eBook, *How to Say No* says when you learn how to assert 'no' with respect, firmly and with compassion, it's likely you'll have others impressed with your self-awareness and class and may even want to be more like you.

Even *Apple* boss, the late Steve Jobs, in one of his seven rules of success outlined in an article in Entrepreneur.com, demonstrates why saying no can have such power. *"When he returned to Apple in 1997, he took a company with 350 products and reduced them to ten products in two years. He was just as proud of what Apple chose not to do."*

Realise now that you cannot do and be it all. As my husband reminds me often, your in-tray will never be empty, so stop burning yourself out by trying to clear it completely.

For me, doing one or two tasks to completion is way more valuable than doing everything mediocre.

I culled those noisy things in my life that were not crucial or serving my core values and got inventive on how to create more time in my day.

You might like to keep in mind the following whether you're saying 'no' to a friend, partner, child, parent, work colleague or boss, to preserve the relationship;

- don't apologise as you are not at fault,
- be polite but firm,
- give a reason but don't make excuses (forget the fluff),
- be honest,
- suggest an alternative, and
- wish them well.

Robyn's recommendations

Think back to those times in your life where you've said 'yes' to something only to feel resentful or drowning under too much to do. What other feelings did you experience and what was the outcome?

Begin being observant of the requests of you and invitations you get, and question if they will move you closer or further away from your goals. Take time to construct a reply if possible so you can practice your saying 'no', gracefully. If you don't have the luxury of having extra time (e.g. if it's a face-to-face request) you can ask for more time and say 'can I get back to you on this' or something to that effect.

CHAPTER 3: KEEPING RECORDS

You can't manage what you can't measure
   Peter Drucker

When you don't make an effort to keep accurate records when attempting a weight loss strategy, you're mostly playing a guessing game. This makes it difficult to do an audit on your current and future eating habits to work towards a desirable outcome and then manage it going forward. This will make your progress and your ultimate end goal a challenge. If you don't have anything to track, you don't have any progress markers to celebrate or work towards. It's the kiss of death to any plans you have for sustaining this journey long-term!

Before we look at the initial steps to *Keeping Records*, I will first share with you:

- why you don't want to omit this crucial part of recording your stats and results.

- And then I'm going to step you through your *Keeping Records* steps:
- **Step 1:** Take your initial weight and body fat percentage (body fat is optional),
- **Step 2:** take your initial body measurements,
- **Step 3:** take your initial photos,
- **Step 4:** start a food journal, and
- **Step 5:** mentally prepare yourself for your start date.

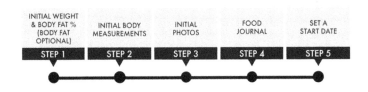

Let's jump right in to understand why you need to commit to the practice of recording your progress.

Recording your results

I cannot stress enough the importance of record keeping throughout this entire process, for both the foods (energy) you consume; *logging*, and the results you achieve along the way; *tracking*.

As the process becomes a little more natural and instinctual, as well as the closer you get to your goal, the level at which you need to take records, log your food and track data may become less and less. But for the initial stages, while you are still finding your feet, it's imperative.

Not only does it help you to see your progression through

the process, but it enables you to see what's working and what may need improving because no two people are the same in the way to approach this *Body Plan*.

Recording your personal data helps you to do a personal audit of your circumstances. As Dr Spencer Nadolsky, American obesity and family doctor promotes, there is a common phenomenon whereby patients think they are diet resistant. But on an investigation, it is determined that what they are eating is far from what they believe themselves to be eating. He doesn't think they're lying per se, but without the actual data, you're just performing a guessing game.

How many times have you finished off your kid's dinner plate or mindlessly snacked while preparing dinner? Every little bit adds up throughout a day, week or year.

In the past I've had some clients resist this part of the process, perhaps they've had a negative attachment to weighing themselves which has triggered obsessive behaviours, or maybe taking the extra few minutes out of their day to track their foods has been a challenge to introduce as a new behaviour. But over time, with this commitment to your planned transformation, you'll be glad you did.

Robyn's recommendation

From the *How to Use This Book* section, you should by now already have your equipment.

You can download your own checklist here in your free starter kit http://bit.ly/bodyplanstarter

Now that you have acquired your equipment, you are ready to start.

Step 1: On waking, take your initial weight and body fat percentage (if possible) after going to the bathroom and preferably naked

 You will be recording your weight and body fat every week on the same day in your calorie tracking smartphone app (*My Fitness Pal* or *Lose It*) and also in your journal. Recording this is necessary for tracking your progress and determining next week's food intake. Ignore the calorie budget the app sets for you as these can often be inaccurate.

Your body fat reading on a scale is not 100 per cent accurate, but nothing is. Water displacement with the body floating in a tank is the best, and that is done in a laboratory and very expensive. However, the scales are useful for comparison measures. These scales measure body fat, and water content in the body by using a low voltage current through you and a scale is developed. You can use them to your advantage by measuring yourself every week at the same time using the same routine up to measuring time. You will get a comparison that may not be 100% accurate, but if you are regular, then the measuring probably will be. These scales may be affected by the water content in your body, so you should try to make your routine dependable.

Step 2: Take your initial body measurements and record these in your journal

Measurements are essential because relying solely on your weight and body fat readings can be inaccurate due to many factors like hormones, the contents of your digestive system, your personal body fat, muscle composition, how hard you are training and your water and carbohydrate intake. During some check-ins, it's possible you may not appear to have lost any weight, you may even seem to gain, but by taking these measurements, you will also be able to determine if you've lost inches/centimetres. This is what occurs when you're losing body fat but retaining muscle. It's smart to have multiple sources of data to measure your progress to keep you motivated.

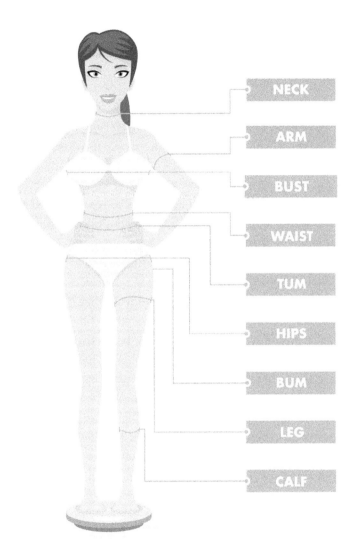

This diagram demonstrates the ideal place to measure. Try to use moles, freckles, birthmarks or other distinguishing marks on your body to ensure that you measure in the same area each time.

Step 3. Take your initial before photos

This is probably the last thing you feel like doing, considering how you most likely think about yourself, but I promise, the satisfaction it will bring you will be worth it, when you look back on your before photo and see how far you have come.

You may not want to have a record of how you look right now, but I guarantee you will be grateful to see your hard work proven both along the way and when you hit your final goal. Hopefully, you won't ever be back here again, so this is your last chance to have some proof of your starting point.

Choose something to wear that's practical to wear every time. Either a bikini or one-piece swimsuit that is form fitting and shows your body, or else workout clothes. The less clothing, the better honestly. Find a place in your house that has plenty of natural sunlight (it's best if the light is shining towards you from a large window) with preferably a very plain background. Take your photos of your front, back and side.

If using a tripod, position the camera at chest height, with enough room in front to take a full body photo. The tripod should be placed precisely square, not from above or below as this will distort your image. If you don't have a tripod for your smartphone (smartphones are best to take photos as they're easy to use and store and view over time – we all have our phones with us most of the time), then ask a trusted loved one to take these photos for you. These photos do not need to be shared with anyone and will be kept entirely private so don't worry about having these as a record. Some smartphones even have apps where you can store all these personal photos in a password protected album that is not visible to anyone except you. I know too many people who've regretted not taking this step – don't be one of them.

Do Steps 1, 2 & 3 weekly at the same time every week

If you prefer you can reduce your progress photos to fortnightly or monthly but don't forget to do them as they are a critical piece of the puzzle. This will be the best way for you to see your progress and you will draw on this data to refine your own individual food intake each week.

Step 4. Start a food journal

For the first week, don't make any drastic adjustments to the way you eat, however, get into the habit of keeping a food journal or recording everything you eat. Even those sneaky leftovers from the kid's plates, the cappuccino you have with your girlfriend or work colleague, last cookie from the packet or the two or three wines you enjoyed after work.

Before you commit to making changes, it's beneficial to do a current audit of your typical eating habits, so then you will have an accurate starting point. So, take the first week to get used to logging and tracking your food intake with very little change to what you usually eat.

If this first week hasn't been a typical week for you due to illness, or an abundance of social events, or something out of the norm, continue logging your food intake for up to two weeks, or wait until you have a typical schedule back in place. The more data you collect, the more precise your goal setting and planning will be moving forward.

As I found with both myself and my coaching clients, this is very eye-opening, and just the awareness and reflection on past habits alone is precious in helping to set the tone for the rest of your transformation.

Many of my clients have lightbulb moments during this exercise, and the self-education they gain is priceless for their road ahead. What many found (and possibly you will too) is that what they usually ate was not even consistent in food choice, quantity or timing, which makes it very difficult to achieve any kind of success or identify what works and what doesn't.

Your food journal or logging is best done using a macro/calorie smartphone app like *My Fitness Pal* or *Lose It* ensuring that you are inputting not only the foods you are eating but how much you're eating, which is where your food scale comes in.

Take care to ensure the foods you select are accurate as there may be many options to choose. So, don't just pick the first one available. For example, random users are able to input their own recipes, ingredients and foods, which mean it is not always accurate in the global database, so don't blindly rely on every input you select. It's up to you to be discerning with your information.

You can always use *Google* to double check the calories and macro data is correct, and you'll find over time you'll usually tend to eat the same foods anyway. So, once you've built up your own data bank, then it will be more relaxed and won't be so time-consuming for you which is one of the reasons people don't stick this part out.

Don't get too caught up on how to log your food in the beginning, just do your best. This phase is just to give you an idea of what your typical eating habits are like, so you've got a starting point. I will cover in more detail what calories and macros mean and how to work out your individual budget further in the book.

Even if you find it difficult to track your current eating habits for a week, completing an introductory food diary of up to two to three days will give you an idea of where you may be sneaking extra snacks or calories in that you hadn't really been aware of.

But understand this now. Logging and tracking your food will form a large part of the ongoing process and will mean the difference between success and mediocrity or even failure. Don't let the uncomfortable feeling that often comes with any form of behaviour change distract you from your ultimate dream. Making peace with this new habit you'll be forming will really help.

For those of us that are parents of young children or even grandparents, finishing off the kid's meals can be a culprit, so too are those sugar dense coffees, cakes or birthday celebrations in the office which can really add up over the day.

The basics of logging and tracking your foods require you to break down your meal into ingredients to be as accurate as possible.

I've attached some examples of my own tracking screenshots from *Lose It*.

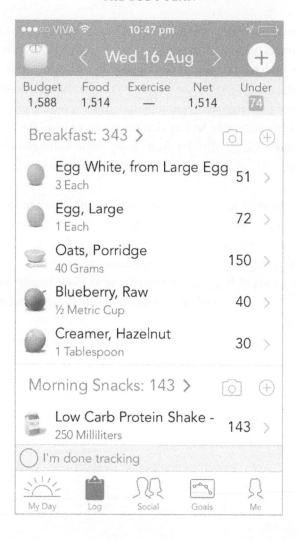

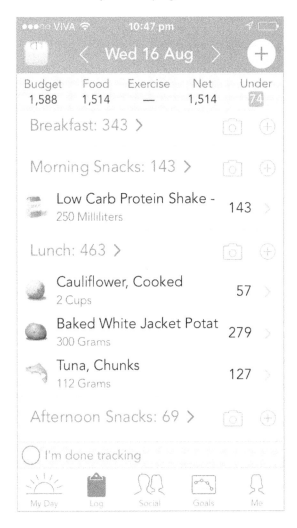

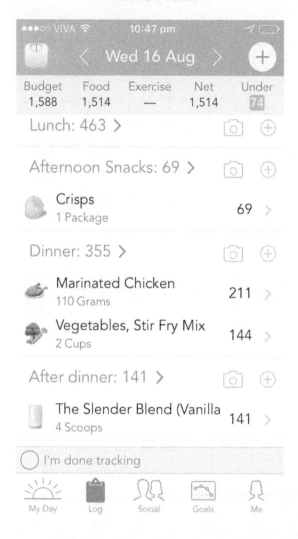

CAN you see how I have recorded not only the foods but the volume too?

Lose It or *My Fitness Pal* will work out the calories but again I will talk to you more about this in *Chapter 4: Understanding Flex-*

ible Dieting. You'll just need to capture your own food diary to look at a typical example of your current dietary habits.

If you are eating packaged food, try out the barcode scanner as most foods can be found there. If not, you can input your own. Just ensure you check the values against the package, and if not correct you can edit them.

Step 5: Mentally prepare yourself for your start date – you're going to need to log and track and measure everything. If you are not measuring, then you have no idea how much you're eating so you cannot control it. Why keep guessing when you can have a scientific and accurate process to follow.

Robyn's recommendations

Before you can really be sold on the success of this plan, you'll need to be committed to taking these first steps and having a starting point no matter how painful it feels to be confronted with some home truths. It's pretty evident in my very own before photo that I wasn't happy with what I saw, but you can bet I was pretty glad I had taken these initial steps in the beginning and now that I'm on the other side of my journey I'm amazed and proud of how far I've come.

PART III

LET'S GET STARTED: FIRST THREE MONTHS

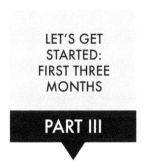

It's possible you jumped straight ahead to this section because you wanted practical steps on what I did get to move towards my dream body, without taking the time to reflect on the foundational work at the beginning of this book.

I will say this; without the understanding that I covered

in *Part II: Foundation Knowledge: Pre-Prep Stage*, your success with *The Body Plan* will be less likely.

There is definitely much work of the mind to be done in the beginning to prepare you for the challenges and journey ahead.

I'd hate for you to give up at the slightest sign of a plateau, or at a social occasion you just can't say no to.

Or cast all dreams away with the notion that you're just too over the hill for this kind of 'radical' change.

By truly understanding what's brought you here to honouring your heart's desire to get healthy, energetic, prevent or delay old age and weight borne ailments, the best chance you have of achieving your goal is just to do the work.

But if you've read through the *Part II: Foundation Knowledge: Pre-Prep Stage* and are now chomping at the bit to embark on your own transformation, then it's time to share it with you right now.

Why are we focusing on just your first three months? Well, what I realised with all my past failed attempts at maintaining a healthy body, fitness and weight level, was that I was focusing on the end goal, and the supposed only temporary lifestyle it was going to take to get me there.

Eventually, I would just give up because the process wasn't sustainable nor enjoyable. Meaning I couldn't see myself having to make the food or lifestyle choices I was required to take, forever. It seemed painful, long and tedious.

As I discussed already, I believe the key to long-lasting success is breaking down your transformation into smaller achievable tasks so that you have adequate time to master each before moving on to the next.

As my own journey progressed, I naturally found three months blocks to be the magic time required to master each phase before proceeding to the next.

Organically, I found in the first twelve months this is what occurred for me:

- **Phase 1 (months 1-3): Nutrition Phase,**
- **Phase 2 (months 4-6): Fitness Phase,**
- **Phase 3 (months 7 -9): Fitness Phase (advanced), and**
- **Phase 4 (months 10 and beyond): Refining Phase (plateaus, getting more efficient with training and nutrition refinements.)**

The first three-month block which I cover in this book should really be focusing on only three main things. They are:

1. Understanding flexible dieting,
2. Planning ahead, and
3. Sustaining your progress.

So, let's dive in, with *Chapter 4: Understanding flexible dieting.*

CHAPTER 4: UNDERSTANDING FLEXIBLE DIETING

Don't be afraid of food. It is fuel – it's the best way to get your ideal physique.

What happens when you're not fully educated in the science behind weight gain and obesity is that you blindly follow random diets that haven't necessarily been created for you and your lifestyle or weight loss goals. Many of these random diets are designed to take your money, often they are misleading and not at all backed by science.

By following the latest fad, you also won't be using your better judgment because you don't know what decisions to make or how to make healthy choices when they're presented to you.

This part of the book will help to give you some necessary, evidence-based and scientific information around food and how to make the healthiest choices for you and your weight loss goals, based on what suits you.

So, what does 'understanding flexible dieting' involve?

- researching and educating yourself on nutrition,
- recognising the value of flexible dieting,
- becoming familiar with basic nutritional biology definitions,
- understanding calories and a calorie deficit,
- knowing your macronutrients and their importance,
- appreciating the need for adequate fibre and hydration,
- calculating your calorie intake, the long and easy way,
- figuring your unique calorie 'budget',
- knowing how to log your food and track your calories,
- reading labels, and
- asking if health foods are really all they're cracked up to be.

Phew! Yep, this is a meaty section so let's dive in, with researching and educating yourself about nutrition.

Become educated

How well do you know your body? It's likely not very well, and that's why you're here now. This is why this transformation will be a total self-discovery: *mind, body* and *soul*. It's time to honour her and the process ahead of you.

There are many layers to what is considered a healthy diet, and it all depends on where you are personally as to where you need to approach it.

It's all good and well to bang on about is your food helping or hindering gut health or are you consuming too much sugar, processed or otherwise, but when it comes to weight loss for those that are not already lean, science says all that matters is that you eat less energy than your body burns off.

Research and educate yourself on science-backed nutrition.

You have to be armed with as much information as possible. You need to invest the time and energy into this if you want to be successful. Be suspicious of fad diets that promise the world.

If the principle of losing weight is to have a calorie deficit as discussed in *Part I: My Philosophy*, the methods to achieve this weight loss can be varied and entirely up to you.

You may elect to eat a high-fat / low carb diet, or you could opt to eat a vegan / plant-based diet. Or as Mark Haub, a professor of human nutrition at *Kansas State University* did, a *Twinkie diet.*

For ten weeks, Haub ate a diet high in processed foods and still lost twenty-seven pounds in two months. All because he kept his calorie intake below his standard daily maintenance budget.

Any particular style of eating will work with regards to weight loss, providing your consumption of calories is less than what your body needs to maintain its weight.

Mark Haub, of the *Twinkie diet* experiment, proved that when it comes to fat loss, calorie counting matters above the nutritional quality of food.

Of course, is the *Twinkie diet* a healthy way to lose weight? That's debatable. However, it was found that as his body fat reduced, so too did his bad cholesterol.

Everyone's caloric needs will be as unique to them as their fingerprints. As I've mentioned earlier, calculating these needs is as much an art as it is a science.

If there were one answer that was the same for everyone,

then it'd be easy. We'd all be walking around with svelte bodies and feeling light and sexy.

But we're not.

Factors that will impact your own dietary needs and calculations are your age, previous diet history, genetics, metabolic health, different backgrounds, life experiences, stressors, emotional and mental hurdles, body type and lifestyle.

Over time, you will get a better understanding of your own body by using the suggesting methods I outline in this book.

Discerning how you personally respond to your new way of eating will take some weeks of monitoring your results, always ensuring you keep accurate records.

Flexible dieting

---

diet1

ˈdʌɪət/

Noun

1. the kinds of food that a person, animal, or community habitually eats. Vegetarian diet synonyms: selection of food, food and drink, food, foodstuffs, provisions, edibles, fare;

2. a special course of food to which a person restricts themselves, either to lose weight or for medical reasons. "I'm going on a diet."

Taken from Google

The term 'diet' gets a bad rap these days, usually because the latter above definition is used more in the mainstream and denotes restriction, adherence, discipline and sometimes unhealthy obsession.

When I refer to *flexible dieting*, it's quite the opposite to what normal conventional diets typically are, which is my definition of torture.

I didn't come up with the term *flexible diet*, but the concept and energy behind it sure seems appropriate to me these days. Particularly after my period as a *raw vegan* which was a very exclusive way of eating.

As the name suggests, the kinds of foods you are able to eat while *flexible dieting* can be adjusted to suit you.

With *flexible dieting*, you are free to construct your diet any way you wish, within a set of broad guidelines.

Flexible dieting allows you to eat what you like and still achieve your body goals.

Depriving yourself in the present moment for a result in the future that may never materialise requires willpower which I've discussed is a finite resource. It's also not something I'm willing to sacrifice, as one of life's joys is the celebration of food. Allowing yourself some enjoyment daily in the foods you eat has been proven to decrease binge eating tendencies and it's much easier to stick to your plan. Be gone, unnecessary food guilt!

Flexible dieting is sometimes called *If It Fits Your Macros* or *IIFYM* for short.

What constitutes a healthy balanced diet is still very contentious, and even researchers can find a result to match their own bias. What I have found to give me a rounded balance of everything I need to feel satisfied is the following based off Alan Aragon, a peer-reviewed nutrition researcher's *10 Essential Characteristics of a Healthy Diet.*

1. A healthy diet respects personal taste preference.

2. A healthy diet provides enough total energy to support physical and mental performance goals, as well as healthy body composition.
3. A healthy diet covers macronutrient and micronutrient needs.
4. A healthy diet has no unnecessary/unfounded food restrictions.
5. A healthy diet respects individual medical intolerances/allergies.
6. A healthy diet is convenient.
7. A healthy diet is affordable.
8. A healthy diet is socially acceptable (and not hazardous to the public).
9. A healthy diet is compatible with personal ideologies.
10. A healthy diet is sustainable in the long-term.

With the *Twinkie diet* my intuition tells me over time the lack of fibre, vitamins and minerals wouldn't be ideal. This is where using the 70/20/10 philosophy as a guideline when constructing your own meal plan as well as the *10 Essential Characteristics of a Healthy Diet* shared above, are going to give you the best all-around version of a sustainable diet, in my opinion.

Nutritional biology definitions

Before we determine your own energy/calorie requirements, you'll need to understand a few of the basic terms used in nutrition biology.

If this is the first time you're seeing the following definitions below, don't panic, it will become clearer over time.

- **Calorie:** is the measurement of energy

- **Maintenance Calories:** the calorie value that your body requires to maintain its current weight
- **Calorie Deficit:** the calorie value that your body requires to be in a weight loss mode
- **Calorie Surplus:** the calorie value that your body requires to be in weight gain mode
- **Macronutrients (Macros):** the breakdown of calories into these macros of protein, carbs and fat (all essential for a healthy functioning system for different reasons)
- **BMR / Base Metabolic Rate:** your base calorie (energy) requirements when you are doing no activity, but your body still continues to pump blood, breath, keep your body functioning at rest, basically keep you alive.

What is a calorie?

It's unlikely that you've never heard of the term *calorie*, but what is it exactly?

In simple terms, it's basically the unit of energy used to describe the energy of any food or drink item. It's a way to describe the power that you intake from consuming this food. In some parts of the world, they prefer the unit of kilojoules which is another way to describe the unit of energy, but for the sake of simplicity, and purely because it's the unit I used while transforming my body, I will only refer to *calories* in this book. If you need to convert to kilojoules, you can look online or use a smartphone app to perform the conversions.

What is a calorie deficit?

A *calorie deficit* essentially means you consume fewer calories (energy) than what your body needs, therefore enabling a shortfall in calories or energy consumption.

Our bodies require energy throughout the day to perform essential functions like pump blood, breathing etc., even when we're not being active. Then add to it the extra strength we require to get out of bed in the morning, walk to the station, go to the supermarket and hit the gym; the more we move, the more energy we require.

When you eat less food than your body spends then your body starts to use its stored fat for energy (fuel), which is where the weight (fat) loss begins to occur.

If you consume more energy than your body needs or uses, then you will be in a *calorie surplus*, and it will store the extra calories (energy) as fat, and you will then gain weight (fat).

And when you ingest the exact number of calories (energy) that your body needs, you are consuming your *calorie maintenance* and you will stay the same weight.

But it's a delicate balance because you don't want to eat too little energy or else your body will start to conserve your energy and make you do things like move less, feel lethargic and possibly slow your metabolism which can make it harder for you to burn or lose fat in the long-term.

So, to work out how much your own unique calorie deficit should be is a bit of trial and error because everyone has a different caloric (energy) need based on so many factors like age, gender, height, current weight. But other factors like previous diet history, genetics, average activity levels, emotional and mental state and even health history can impact your own specific needs. I'll show you how to do this further in this chapter.

Macronutrients

Eating within your calorie budget will help you lose weight but breaking down your foods into the three macronutrients and aiming to hit these targets is the next level in the hierarchy of importance.

Macronutrients are *protein, carbohydrates & fat* (and some consider *alcohol* to be the fourth macronutrient which I will discuss more in *Chapter 5: Planning Ahead).*

Protein is required in your diet for muscle building and growth, repair and maintenance.

Carbohydrates give you the energy to get through your day as your body's primary source of energy.

And good dietary fat is used as building blocks of the human body and is essential for hormone health.

And *alcohol*, well it's just fun. I'll discuss this later.

Although it's not the most crucial component to your weight loss plan, ideally once you've got a good handle on your caloric needs, then working out your daily macronutrient requirement is next in importance.

Aiming for a balanced macronutrient meal will help you to retain muscle while your body is mostly in a degenerative mode, reduce your risk of hunger, give you adequate energy so you don't get brain fog, and ensure your hormones are being looked after. How you construct your macronutrient balance won't impact weight loss, because as we already know, a calorie deficit is all you need to do that, but it will make all the difference with how you feel. Diets that require you to eliminate or severely reduce a macronutrient, like the *Atkins* (low carb high protein) or *ketogenic* (high-fat, low carb) diets, often come with an adjustment period. For example, whenever I've reduced my carbs to very low, I have had an extremely fuzzy head and low energy. Keep it balanced is my motto and it's what has worked. The balance may be different from you to me, as you may favour more fat than carbs than I, but the beauty is you don't have to stick to it every day.

I'll show you how to get an idea of a balanced meal and macronutrients further in this chapter.

Macronutrient values

You won't need to know this information verbatim, especially if you are using an automatic calorie tracker/manager or an app, but it's important to know what value your macronutrients carry.

1g protein = 4 calories

1g of carbohydrates = 4 calories

1g of fat = 9 calories

1g of alcohol = 7 calories

You can see that both carbs and proteins have the same calorie value per gram; however, fat is a higher source of energy per gram.

If you opt to eat more fat than carbs in your diet, just understand that the volume of food you will be able to eat will be less before you hit your calorie limit.

Low-fat foods may be higher in carbs (sugar is often added to render the food more palatable when the fat is taken away), which is ok if it brings down the calorie content of your diet, but just be mindful of this when you start to design your own meal planner.

Fibre

I never truly appreciated the value of fibre until embarking on this body transformation.

As a raw vegan in days gone by, my diet was abundant in

fibre without me even realising it, from my morning green smoothie chock full of vegetables and fruit to my lunchtime meal-sized salads and my plant filled dinners. Being regular was never an issue.

With the variety allowed in *flexible dieting*, however, it's worth noting that fibre, or the lack thereof, will let you know soon enough.

The purpose of fibre in our diet is as our intestinal broom. It aids in the removal of waste and pushes our toxins outside in the form of a stool.

Fibre is the part of plant foods that cannot be digested or absorbed and stored in the body.

Back in my juicing days, it was easy to see what fibre actually was. It is the waste part of the fruits and vegetables that are left behind once all the juicy goodness is extracted. It's believed this juice is absorbed directly into the body because the fibre is removed.

This is the premise behind juicing being very quick for the body to assimilate the nutrients because there is no fibre for the body to break down when consumed. The fibre slows down the digestion process. The juicer essentially does the breaking down for you.

Despite the ability for us to lose weight eating a *Twinkie diet* or any other kind of processed food, your overall health will begin to suffer over time if you don't aim to hit a minimum daily target of fibre.

I don't need to really monitor my fibre intake too closely these days, as my diet is mostly balanced, but my body will tell me when I have consumed too little or too much.

Too little is usually after an extremely social weekend, eating more processed foods with very little fruit or vegetables, which tends to leave me feeling either clogged up or a little gassy.

On the other hand, being a little over-enthusiastic with your fibre consumption can ensure you're super cleaned out if you get my drift.

Other benefits of adequate fibre in your daily diet are feelings of satiety and fullness which is fantastic when aiming to have a calorie deficit.

Foods that are higher in fibre:

- vegetables,
- fruits,
- grain products: like pasta, bread, oats, rice (wholegrain has higher fibre as the refining process strips the outer bran reducing fibre content),
- beans, peas and other legumes, and
- nuts and seeds.

Robyn's recommendation

The *British Nutrition Organisation* suggests the following guidelines for fibre intake and states that it's likely most people are probably only reaching approximately 18g per day.

AGE (YEARS)	RECOMMENDED INTAKE OF FIBRE
2-5	15 grams per day
5-11	20 grams per day
11-16	25 grams per day
17 and over	30 grams per day

You can achieve this by:

- starting the day with a high fibre breakfast like oats, or high fibre cereal,
- adding extra or increasing your vegetable servings with your main meals,
- enjoying a side salad with the main meal,
- opting for wholegrain over white products (although the calorie values rarely differ),
- enjoying fruits and vegetable with the skins, (potatoes, pumpkins, apples etc.),
- eating fruit for snacks,
- blending hidden green leafy vegetables (like kale) to your protein shake, and
- grating zucchini into cooked dishes.

These are several suggestions you can employ to increase your daily fibre intake.

Hydration

I think we all know by now that drinking water is essential for overall health function but determining the correct required for optimal health and weight loss per day is debatable.

It's estimated we exhale two cups a day as water vapour and our bodies require approximately six cups a day for general functioning, add in another two cups that gets sweated out if you're in a hot climate or exercising. Add a couple more cups for weight loss, and you're already at approximately ten cups of water minimum that you should be drinking per day.

As for aiding your weight loss, drinking water is calorie free, can help to curb appetite, especially if you're between meals and can increase energy.

Hunger can also be mistaken for true thirst as well, so it's important you stay hydrated, especially when you're in weight loss mode.

Dehydration can also cause you to retain fluid which makes you feel and sometimes look bloated and can give you a false impression of your weight loss success, by showing a higher scale reading which isn't fat, but water weight.

It sounds counter-intuitive, but drinking more water helps to reduce and flush out fluid retention. Another great reason to drink more water.

Robyn's recommendation

Take note of your daily water consumption and increase it if necessary, aiming for between two and three litres a day.

Calculate your daily calorie needs for weight loss

The Easy Way – Skip this section if you'd prefer to use my own online calculator that will work this out for you automatically.

**You can access my own online calculator here on my website
http://bit.ly/bodyplancalc**

The Longer Way – As the name suggests takes longer, and you don't really need to do it this way, but I've included this for those, like me, who want to learn more.

The calculations I share are using common industry accepted formulas that are based on averages. Some are more accurate than others, but as with most biological formulas, it's impossible to generate an exact answer for you.

We just use this as a starting point for you, and monitor your results moving forward.

Personal activity levels are always subjective, rarely ever

exact from one day to another, and everybody responds differently to various forms of exercise.

Depending on your body composition and other general factors, these will impact your very own initial calculation, please take your answers with a grain of salt as they are just to get you started.

After a few weeks of accurate tracking and record management, you'll be able to learn more about your own personal responses to the energy you consume and how much your body needs. The most important thing here is aiming for consistency; of record keeping and adhering to your targets each week.

As well as logging and tracking your results from week-to-week, other well-being self-check assessments I'd suggest you monitor and keep a record in your journal of are your:

- moods,
- energy levels,
- experiencing cravings for particular types of foods,
- sleep / rest,
- menstrual cycle,
- injuries, and
- fitness / strength.

The above will help you to reconcile when you're eating too little, what triggers certain eating habits, what kind of exercise is suitable for you and more.

Every little bit of information you can record helps you to become a bit more self-aware and propel you forward on this transformation road.

If you prefer to use an online self-check assessment, you can access mine here in your free starter kit:
http://bit.ly/bodyplanstarter

There are free and paid applications, software and services available to help you calculate your own budget, but I'd suggest you use my very own online calculator as I mentioned earlier.

Please note: I don't recommend using *My Fitness Pal* or *Lose It's* inbuilt calorie budget calculator as their results are often inaccurate.

The best way to really get to know your own personal budget is to do these initial calculations and then monitor your progress from week-to-week to see how your own body responds.

If you're like me too, you like to understand 'the why' not just 'the how', so even if you do choose to use my calculator after you've read this part, I want to share this with you, so you'll have a greater understanding of how the formula is worked out.

Now you have an understanding of the underlying biological terms and definitions, you will be able to create your own starting point.

One of the best ways to appreciate how this works is to imagine that you've allocated yourself a daily spend of money to buy your food.

You can either blow it all on one decadent gourmet meal that will taste delicious but might make you feel hungry for the rest of the day

OR

Divide your budget across four to five meals over the day, balancing your meals with palatable lower calorie, highly nutritious foods that will help you feel fuller for longer

OR

Divide your spending over two to three larger meals that will more satisfying than smaller but more frequent meals but will be a longer window of time between meals (great for those who rely on meal breaks at work or don't enjoy eating smaller more frequent meals).

Then once that bank account has been emptied for that day

you are out of cash until it resets the following day. Once your money is gone, it's gone.

How to calculate your daily calorie budget

Before we can determine how many calories a day you should eat to lose weight, we need first to understand what your own maintenance calories are and to do so, as a starting point, we'll need to use a biological formula.

In the beginning, calculating your maintenance calories this way isn't 100 per cent accurate, because, like most biological formulas, they are understood to be generic only. It's impossible to know precisely for sure what each and every person's specific calorie requirements are because we all have different body composition, (muscle to fat ratio) diet and health profiles. However, with some of your personal historical data under your belt from accurate record keeping over time, you will become more self-aware of your own body's needs which will help with your weight loss goals.

Before we can calculate your *daily calorie* targets to lose weight, we first need to understand what your *maintenance calorie* targets are. Before we can calculate your *maintenance calorie* targets, we must first determine what your *basal metabolic rate (BMR)* is.

For this calculation, I favour the *Harris-Benedict Equation,* to first calculate your *BMR.*

Step 1. Calculate your *BMR*
Harris Benedict Equation

Example: A woman who is 40 years old, 173cm and 75kg:
$$BMR = 655.1 + (9.563 \times \text{weight in kg}) + (1.850 \times \text{height in cm}) -$$
$$(4.676 \times \text{age in years})$$
Basal metabolic rate = 1505

BMR Calculation for Women	(metric) BMR=665.1 + (9563 x weight in kg) + (1.850 x height in cm) - (4.676 x age in years)
	(imperial) BMR=665.1 + (4.35 x weight in pounds) + (4.7 x height in inches) - (4.7 x age in years)
BMR Calculation for Men	(metric) BMR=66.5 + (13.75 x weight in kg) + (5.003 x height in cm) - (6.76 x age in years)
	(imperial) BMR=66 + (6.2 x weight in pounds) + (12.7 x height in inches) - (6.76 x age in years)

Step 2. Calculate your *Maintenance Calorie Budget*

Now you have determined your own *BMR*, you can now calculate your *maintenance calorie* budget.

We are trying to find your starting point and also because I've previously mentioned to not focus on fitness for the first one to three months, I would suggest you use the *None* or *Light* activity levels calculations, just to begin with.

This is because we are trying to get the most accurate start point for you as possible and moving forward this may or may not change.

This result will give you the approximate daily *calorie budget* you should aim for if you wish to maintain your current weight (*maintenance calories*).

But you're most likely wanting to lose weight, isn't that why you're reading this book? So, we now need to calculate your calorie deficit budget.

Calculations are:

- None / little to no exercise = BMR x 1.2
- Light / exercise/sports 1-3 days a week = BMR x 1.375
- Moderate / moderate exercise/sports 3-5 days a week = BMR x 1.55
- Active / hard exercise/sports 6-7 days a week = BMR x 1.725
- Very Active / very intense exercise/sports & physical occupation and/or weight lifting 2-3 a week = BMR x 1.9

Example: 75kgs and BMR = 1505
None/little to no exercise = 1505 x 1.2 = 1806
Maintenance calories are 1806

Step 3. Calculate your *Calorie Deficit Budget*
Maintenance Budget x 0.85 = your Daily Calorie Budget

Example: 1806 x 0.85 = 1535
Calorie deficit budget = 1535 calories per day

Step 4. Calculate your *Daily Protein Goal*

Calorie management is king when it comes to losing weight, but if you want to focus on reducing mostly fat and retain as much muscle as possible while helping to ensure that you feel fuller for longer, then hitting your daily protein target should be of importance to you. Eating adequate protein will help you to look leaner and toned, and when you eat protein, it's much harder for your body to store it as unwanted fat so the more you eat, the better for your fat loss goals.

Calculations are:

Daily protein goal (metric)
Weight in kg x 1.8

Example: 75kg x 1.8 = 135
Daily protein goal = 135g per day

Daily protein goal (imperial)
Weight in lbs x 0.81

Example: 165lbs x 0.81 = 135
Daily protein goal = 134g per da

Step 5. Calculate your *Daily Minimum Fat Goal*

Many people who've had a history of dieting may be fearful of eating fat, or on the other hand with the recent trend of ketogenic diets, you may be consuming fat by the gallon.

The role fat plays in our diet is a significant one, so don't be shy in consuming it, but just remember, fat, unlike protein and carbs has a higher calorie content per volume, so it's easier to overshoot your calorie budget when you eat a higher fat diet.

There is a sweet spot between still enjoying fat which has an added benefit of making you feel fuller for longer and overindulging, so don't go too crazy on the low-fat foods, but don't take this as permission to eat as much fat as you want. You may find yourself getting to midday and having no more calories left in your food budget for the day if you're not careful.

I like to use a rule of thumb to aim for 25 to 30 per cent of your calorie intake as fat, but this will be a personal preference.

It's advisable to never go as low as 15 per cent of your total calories as fat.

<u>Calculations are:</u>

(Calorie deficit budget x 0.3) / 9 = your daily minimum fat in grams.

Example: a 75kg person
(1535 x 0.3) / 9 = 51g of fat
Daily calorie intake of fat minimum = 51g

Robyn's recommendation

If these manual calculations have lost you, don't worry, all you need to do is use my free online calculator – it will take all the thinking out of it for you.

**You can access my own online calculator here on my website
http://bit.ly/bodyplancalc**

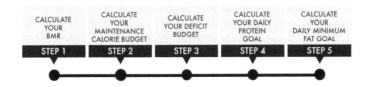

Now you have a starting point with which to create your week's eating plan which I will cover in *Chapter 5: Planning Ahead.*

Logging your food intake

Logging (or recording) your food intake is going to be the difference between success and failure. Why guess when you can know for sure how much you can eat?

Despite some people's resistance to doing this for fear of becoming obsessed or anxious with their intake, it's really just an accurate way to perform a self-audit on your behaviours around food as well as data collection to understand what your body needs and wants to function as healthy as possible. It's a smart way to understand portion control. The thing is, we all need energy (food) in the very least to stay alive and we all need even more strength to be active, however, if we over-consume, we gain weight.

How do I suggest determining the difference between adequate energy or over consumption?

Logging your daily intake enables us to understand where

we're going right and wrong and be strategic and fully in control of our body's needs. This will help to ensure you don't over-eat (weight gain) or under-eat (risk of bingeing when your intake gets too low).

How to log your food

Depending on whether keeping a food diary or recording your intake is entirely a new concept to you or not, or if you've tried *logging* in the past but soon tired of it, will really impact how you attack this part of the process.

If you are entirely new to *logging* your food, at this stage I will encourage a gentle and flexible approach that will see you taking it one step at a time, building your confidence and practice, so you don't overwhelm yourself and give up at the first sign of resistance.

Often, it's just the first step of doing this work that is the challenge, but once you make it part of your typical day, it will feel more natural and become quicker. You will find as time goes by, you won't need to be this vigilant.

1. Familiarise yourself with any of my suggested calorie smartphone apps as mentioned in the *How to Use This Book: Before You Get Started: Equipment Required.* You can download your own equipment checklist in your free starter kit http://bit.ly/bodyplanstarter. The apps are pretty straightforward when it comes to using them but allow yourself time to get to know how it works and what information it will collect on both the free and paid versions. Personally, I do prefer *Lose It* over *My Fitness Pal,* and I have paid for the premium version as it offers more insights and the ability to modify your planning and functionality to plan ahead of time. At the time of publishing, *My Fitness Pal* does seem to be more robust if you're looking for a more comprehensive app. The reasons I prefer *Lose It* are I

prefer the interface and usability, it's simpler to use and has less complexity, and adding food seems to be faster.

2. Add each food item one by one, per ingredient, being as accurate as possible, realising that if you input oats or yoghurt for example, across brands the values can be very different. When adding in foods like waffles or pancakes, I'd suggest you insert the whole recipe into the database then portion off how much you consumed. Usually by weight or quantity of said food. If it's a recipe you'll regularly be using, once you spend the extra time initially to input into your database, you'll be able to use it time and time again. I show you how to log recipes in *Chapter 5: Planning Ahead.* For other simpler inputs, I do prefer to add in each food item individually as opposed to random recipes or multiple ingredient foods that are already in the database which aren't always verified. For whole and natural foods like fruits, eggs and vegetables you can either input them by weight or quantity.

3. Play around with working out if *logging* your future intake, a day ahead, works better for you, or if you prefer being more spontaneous and *logging* your food as you eat it. In most cases, I plan my following day's meals ahead of time (usually when I'm lying in bed with my five-year-old at bedtime). I find the days I don't do this, and I'm winging it, I tend to get to the end of the day and I'm stuck. I'm either trying to play catch up with calorie and macro Tetris to compile my last meal of the day, or I'm annoyed with myself for having no calories left and still being hungry. At least by planning my meals ahead of time, I allow less room for error and take the decision making out of my following day, which helps mental bandwidth for other more important things. It also helps with my bulk meal preparations. Remember I discussed reducing decision fatigue in Part I, the section on *Mind*?

4. Add your foods either manually by searching the database

or inputting in your own single ingredients. If you are eating processed foods with a barcode, often you'll be able to find the food in the database by scanning the barcode or even typing in the brand in the extensive search area. Just make sure you verify the calories and macronutrients on the back of the packets to ensure they're correct, as recipes can change, or be improved, or user inputs can be incorrect. I talk more about the importance of reading labels further in this chapter. Also, a food listing in the databases may be verified by the company as being accurate if it has some type of a checkmark, but it's not always monitored.

5. Be discerning of your inputs. Calorie tracker apps do their best to ensure the nutrition information for foods accurately reflects nutrition information from the product packaging; however, you can imagine how big a job it would be to police, especially when many of the foods in their databases are created by users. According to *Lose It*, even with a verified checkmark, occasionally food will have nutrition information inaccuracies. They are always working to improve the accuracy of nutrition information for foods, and new foods are being added all the time. What I did way back at the beginning of my journey was to schedule extra time to double check my own inputs against *Google*, if there were multiple sources in the database. And from then on in, I always use the same foods, as I tend to eat similar foods on repeat. I do now and again double check my inputs just in case recipes have changed.

6. Not only are you *logging* all the types of foods you are consuming, but also the portion of your meals. If you don't keep score on the volume of each food item, then how do you hope to manage it? This is where your food scale is going to come in, which I talk more about in *Chapter 5: Planning Ahead*.

7. Eating out will make *logging* and tracking a little more challenging, but not impossible. It's better to input something rather than nothing, and over time of eating more foods at

home, you'll become more confident with portion sizes and how much food you need to feel satisfied. I will share more tips and guidance on eating out in *Chapter 5: Planning Ahead*.

8. Don't leave anything out. If you are polishing off the kids' plates or coming home hungry after a morning of errands and happen to eat a handful of Oreos in haste, *log* it. It still counts. If you're mindlessly nibbling on nuts at the bar, or picking at some starters at a party, include it. And if you know you're over-eating, or making poorer than normal choices, *log* it too. Ever little bit of data helps tell a story. The more information you have, the better equipped you'll be to understand your own body and your behaviours and relationship with food. Over time, you'll discover that you tend to eat the same brands and food types, so don't despair in the beginning with the extra time it takes to *log* them; it will become a lot quicker over the coming weeks and months.

9. Don't include any exercise calories earned as some apps will allow you to sync with a heart rate monitor or a *Fitbit*. Don't count exercise as a way to 'earn' back calories. We are focusing purely on input (food intake) not output (activity) in this phase. There is room for exercise in a healthy lifestyle, but as mentioned in *Phase I*, we are focusing on building healthy eating habits first. The technology just doesn't exist to report the calories you can earn from exercise accurately.

!! Warning!!

Once you've determined your daily *calorie* budget, it might feel tempting to undercut this amount of food, to expedite your weight loss. I want to caution you against this. It's super important to know that while you are aiming to be in a *calorie deficit* during your weight loss phase, if you consume too little calories and are below your unique *BMR*, even if you do lose weight, your body will be placed under extreme stress. If you go too low-calorie, you are likely to use muscle as well as fat for energy, meaning if you do lose weight during this time, you may become thinner but have no tone. Your body's desire to move will become less, with a feeling of lethargy, and what's more, you may even damage your metabolism as it slows to reduce your activity levels to conserve your energy.

Damaging your metabolism is definitely not a good idea because a healthy metabolic rate is what you need to burn calories in your everyday life. You don't want to be always in diet-mode, and this is what restricting yourself too much can do in the long-term.

Going below your *BMR* rate for any period is not what your body wants or needs. As I've talked about previously, your *BMR* is what your body needs just to function and to go beneath this can cause damage that will set your goals back.

You can still safely lose weight without causing your metabolism or body to be under unwanted stress. We want to be kind to your body, not hurt it further.

Also eating fewer calories than your body needs, over time, will increase your risk of over-eating, and if you are exercising, your recovery will suffer and take it from someone who knows, you won't be a charming person to be around.

Reading labels

Reading labels is going to become your sport of choice at the beginning of your journey.

I remember thinking back to the start of my very own journey, wondering why I would need to learn how to read labels when I intended to eat all and only whole and natural foods anyway, nothing that came in a packet. But you'd be surprised how difficult that is to do and impractical as well because I don't live in a vacuum.

And as time went by, what I was eating and the real value of energy in my Greek yoghurt or a couple of slices of cheese on crisp-bread became so much easier to appreciate.

The thing is, when you aim to be perfect, you'll be disappointed, so appreciate that there are going to be moments that you will be eating processed food and not allowing yourself to feel guilty about it, will ensure your success.

Example:

Typically, the foods I tend to eat most that have labels are:

- **breakfast:** oats, pre-made salsa, bacon, bread,
- **morning tea:** protein powder,
- **lunch:** low carb and conventional wraps and tortillas, pre-made salsa, bought salad dressing, tuna in a can,
- **afternoon tea:** rice cakes, yoghurt, chocolate, sugar-free sweetener, and
- **dinner:** butter on my vegetables or baked potato, any sauces or seasonings that I add to my dinners etc.

Getting into the habit of reading labels and understanding food calorie and macro values will really give you the edge on your transformation.

Sometimes foods are marketed as 'healthier' or 'high protein', and they're not compared to something else that has a better nutritional profile. Some are even labelled as low-fat, but the calories are much higher than the full-fat version because they've added so much more sugar to make the food more palatable.

This is really a challenging chapter to write for everyone to appreciate because the way you design your own personal menu will differ from person to person. Everyone has varied food preferences, but an example of where I make a concerted effort to read labels is with my Greek yoghurt, which is a staple in my daily diet to ensure I am getting adequate protein. You can only eat chicken breasts or tins of tuna just so many times.

Greek yoghurt is delicious, and I can buy it plain and add my own additions to it, buy it flavoured, or even add it to my savoury meals like a burrito bowl or a lentil soup.

One brand I buy doesn't mention anything about being high in protein but is 0 per cent fat.

Another brand I buy is labelled as low-fat and high protein.

When you compare them side by side, the first brand is much higher protein than the one that is marketed as high protein.

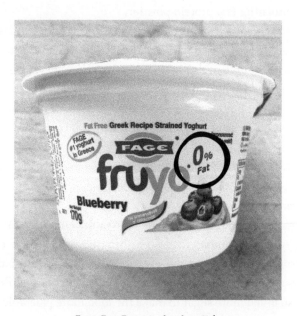

Front: Fage Fruyo marketed as 0% fat

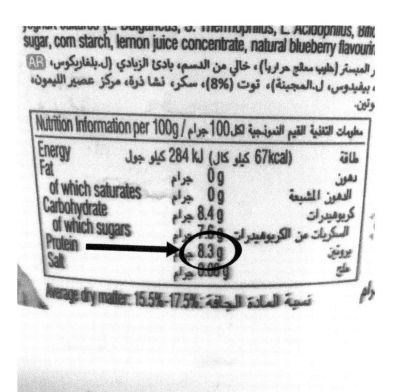

Back: 8.3g of protein per 100g, however the front of the
package is not promoting it's high protein state, rather that it
is 0% fat

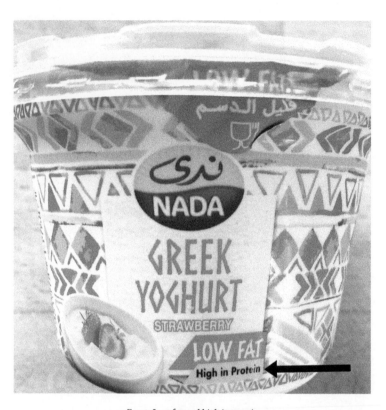

Front: Low fat and high in protein

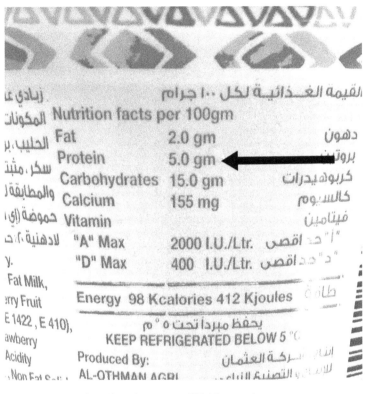

Back: 5g of protein per 100g, which is less protein per gram
compared to the Fage Fruyo despite being marketed as high
in protein

Another example is the bread tortilla wraps I buy that are sold as low carb. When I looked at the labels side by side with the regular wraps, the calorie content is not much different.

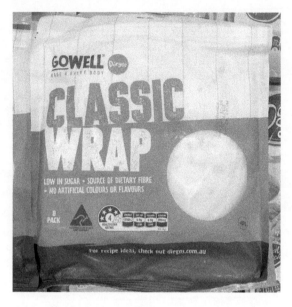

Front

NUTRITIONAL INFORMATION

Servings per package: 8 | Serving size: 50g

	Ave Qty per Serve	Ave Qty per 100g
Energy	625 kJ	1250 kJ
Protein	3.6 g	7.2 g
Fat - Total	4.0 g	8.0 g
- Saturated	0.5 g	0.9 g
Carbohydrate	23.1 g	46.1 g
- Sugars	0.4 g	0.8 g
Dietary Fibre	2.6 g	5.1 g
Sodium	198 mg	395 mg

Back: Classic wrap = 625kj / 149 calories per wrap

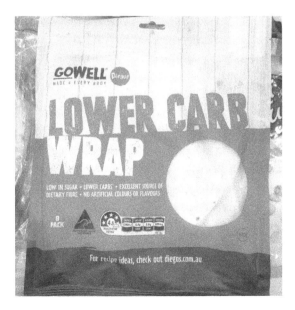

Front

NUTRITIONAL INFORMATION
Servings per package: 8 | Serving size: 50g

	Ave Qty per Serve	Ave Qty per 100g
Energy	692 kJ	1380 kJ
Protein	3.4 g	6.9 g
Fat - Total	4.3 g	8.6 g
- Saturated	0.4 g	0.8 g
Carbohydrate	15.2 g	30.3 g
- Sugars	1.4 g	2.8 g
Dietary Fibre	16.0 g	31.9 g
Sodium	314 mg	628 mg

Back: Lower carb wrap = 692kj / 165 calories. Lower carb doesn't always mean lower calorie.

Sure, the macros are much lower in carbs for the wraps, but in this instance sometimes I will select the regular tortilla just because they taste much better. On the other hand, tortilla wraps can vary significantly in calorie content, so when you start getting more comfortable with reading labels and selecting brands you prefer, you will be able to see where the sneaky calories have been adding up to hinder your weight loss goals.

Health foods

In my previous life as a high-raw foodist (that meant I followed a vegan and predominantly raw food vegan diet), I held the firm belief that it didn't matter how much food I ate – as long as it was mostly raw and vegan I would be the epitome of health. I also believed that as a side effect of this holy grail of health, I would not gain any excess weight or if I was carrying extra weight it would normalise to my ideal weight.

This theory held true for me for the first couple of years that I practised this lifestyle, however after I became a mother and I returned to that way of eating for a brief time, I struggled to lose my post-baby weight, and it actually began to increase.

At the time I really couldn't understand why. Weren't green smoothies holier-than-thou? Açaí bowls, the quintessential breakfast? Raw cashew cheesecakes free from guilt?

Well, it depends. If your goal is weight loss, your body doesn't discriminate against 'health' foods or junk. It just recognises the energy from the foods and decides whether to store it or use it for fuel depending on how much you consume.

Since learning more about the science behind weight loss (energy in, energy out) it doesn't matter if what you're eating is organic, cold-pressed, natural or whole foods. If you're eating more than your body burns off, it's going to store it as fat.

In recent years, we've become obsessed with healthy living, organic, antibiotic free, superfoods, you-name-it, and more in our quest for ultimate health and the impossible immortality.

The number of times I've had friends and clients tell me that they're baffled as to why:

- the coconut oil they've added to their coffee,
- the handful of activated almonds or cashews they're snacking on,
- the afternoon brownie they've replaced with a raw nut-based dessert,
- the cashew milk they're drinking by the gallon, or
- the whole avocado they're enjoying at breakfast,

isn't resulting in their desired weight loss are too many to count.

Just like with learning to read labels, overconsumption of healthy foods or foods marketed as such will still result in weight gain.

Don't be fooled by the term healthy. Even a chicken salad can be more calories than a beef burger. Every Thursday afternoon, as is my current ritual with my kids, we head to our local rugby club for soccer and netball training. As it's the end of the working and school week here in Bahrain, we celebrate with me not having to cook dinner and the kids choosing their favourite take away meal. I indulge with them and often enjoy the club's delicious barbecue beef burger. One week I really felt like ordering their chicken Moroccan salad with quinoa and tangy dressing. Afterwards, when I tallied up the calories, the salad far outshone the beef burger by an extra 250 calories. Even the chicken breast burger is 50 calories more than the beef burger because the chicken breast is double the size of the beef burger patty.

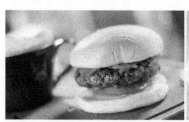 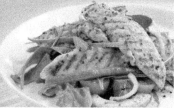

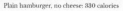

Plain hamburger, no cheese: 330 calories

Grilled chicken salad with couscous, avocado & lemon dressing: 580 calories

So, for the purposes of weight loss success, and your own self-monitoring it's imperative you appreciate that eating all the avocado might help your skin and nails radiate, but over-eating it will not result in you hitting your goal. This is the benefit of tracking and logging all foods you intake.

Robyn's recommendation

Understanding *flexible dieting* is really the crux of *The Body Plan*, but don't let the dryness of this chapter scare you off. Once you really grasp all of this science, you will find it becomes familiar and then automatic, and then you'll be off and racing towards your ideal body in no time.

CHAPTER 5: PLANNING AHEAD

Know what your week is going to look like before you even begin. It's hard to score when you don't have a goal. Never start your week without a plan in mind.

What happens when you don't plan ahead? Well, when you fail to plan, you plan to fail. Which would you prefer? To maintain a healthy weight and lifestyle, or to be back on the yo-yo bandwagon? Need I say any more?

There are some tasks you need to work through when it comes to being well organised *on The Body Plan*, and they include:

Designing your meal plan:

- **Step 1: decide on your meal frequency,**
- **Step 2: forecast the calorie value of each meal, and**
- **Step 3: create your ideal day/week menu plan by:**

- selecting your favourite and neutral tasting foods,

- following meal planning guidelines,
- taking advantage of extra flavour enhancers,
- choosing lower calorie but high flavour food swaps,
- understanding foods labelled 'diet',
- reading my thoughts on cheat meals,
- recognising your trigger foods,
- preparing meals, the easy way,
- managing hunger and ensuring adequate food volume,
- learning how to control your intake and make it part of your day,
- learning how to handle logging food when eating away from home,
- logging and tracking multiple-serve recipes when cooking for more than one,
- understanding the difference between units and quantity,
- eating mindfully and knowing how to use a visual portion guide,
- dealing with alcohol,
- knowing the difference between macros and calories and which is more important,
- thinking of meal prep and planning, especially with a family that won't be eating the same way, and
- looking at my very own sample meal plan and a few of my favourite go-to recipes.

So, let's get started with designing your meal plan.

Design your meal plan

Now that you have your very own calorie and macronutrient budget, you can get to work planning and managing your intake.

Depending on what kind of person you are, whether you thrive on routine and prefer to eat at the same time every day (which can most definitely help with eliminating decision fatigue and ensuring new healthy habits are formed), or you prefer to be more spontaneous, the beauty in this way of eating is very adaptable.

My recommendation, in the beginning, is to have very little wiggle room for error and be as compliant to my suggestions as possible. Because this is how it worked best for me. Over time as you relearn how to eat again, it will become second nature, and you will know how to troubleshoot and manoeuvre through these new changes to your routine.

As Barry Schwartz wrote about in his 2004 book, *The Paradox of Choice: Why More is Less,* the more options you have, the less likely you are to make a choice.

Try to keep every day or most days to this routine as best as you can. There will always be days here and there that will make it difficult to adhere to your plan, but in the beginning, if you can do it more often than not, it will help to set you up going forward.

The way to do this is as follows:

Step 1: decide on your meal frequency

Some prefer to eat three more substantial meals, with more time between meals, others enjoy eating and look forward to eating every two to three hours. Just know whatever you decide will impact how frequently you need to sit down to eat. Preferably choose a plan that you can maintain on weekdays and week-ends. For example, if you have set meal breaks for work and are unable to eat on the job, then you will need to design your meal plan around it.

For myself, I planned to eat five meals a day because my

previous eating habits had been somewhat irregular, and I really needed to reprogram from over-eating when starving or grabbing convenient foods. I liked the idea of eating every two to three hours to further instil automation and habit-stacking.

So, for me, this looked like:

Meal 1: breakfast 630am,
Meal 2: morning tea 930/10am,
Meal 3: lunch 130/2pm,
Meal 4: afternoon tea 4pm, and
Meal 5: Dinner 6pm.

After a few weeks my desire to eat became timely and automatic, and for the first time in many years I would wake up hungry, looking forward to my breakfast. My body was becoming a well-functioning machine, often reminding me of an upcoming meal time around twenty to thirty minutes prior with a little grumble. It was fascinating.

Step 2: now that you've decided on your meal frequency, you will need to forecast the calorie value of each meal

Again, this is a personal preference and one that you're bound to refine and tweak over time. You can decide if you want your meals to be approximately of equal value and portion size, or if you'd rather have larger meals and smaller snacks. Perhaps you would prefer to eat light during the day and enjoy a more substantial dinner at night.

My meals initially, and even to this day, resemble very similar portion and energy value sizes across the day.

I basically took my daily calorie budget and divided by five.

Your daily calorie budget / your meal frequency = your average meal calorie allowance.
Example: 1500 calories / 5 = 300 calories per meal

Of less importance but still valid to know and work out, is roughly how much protein you should aim for at every meal. This is something I don't get too concerned about in this initial phase, but it will help to give you a ballpark figure to aim towards and improve on each week.

For example, if my daily protein goal is 130g over five meals, I should aim for about 26g of protein at each meal. This is not always the same, as my breakfasts tend to be extremely high protein compared to my lunch, but having something to shoot for at each meal helps me to construct a well-balanced and satisfying meal.

To make this calculation easier for you, I've created a simple to use online meal planning calculator you can access here on my website http://bit.ly/bodyplancalc

I don't worry so much about the fats and carbohydrates balanced out over each meal, because I find the carbs and fats are naturally drawn into my diet when I include whole foods like vegetables, fruits, bread, pasta and rice and fats like avocado, bacon, cheese and olive oil.

Step 3: design your ideal day/week menu plan

This part is crucial and cannot be overlooked if you truly want results. Honestly, when I say that you really need these three months to hone and automate your meal planning and preparation, I really mean it. This is where you have the benefit of now having more free time as you are no longer focusing on your fitness during this period, and you've created the space and cleared or reduced the chaos in your life.

I remember sitting down to do this some mornings after school drop off with the kids, where I would typically be running errands or hitting the gym, and it really did take some time to set the groundwork.

I recall thinking, geez, is this really going to take so much of my day? But like anything, once the hard work is done, you should be able to eat and repeat, and over time it's never been easier, saving me from decision fatigue and giving me the equivalent of more hours in my day.

Here's how to get started:

Look at the supplied list of proteins, carbohydrates and fats and select those that you like the taste of, or that are neutral to your palate.

I've provided an online checklist that you can access here in your free starter kit http://bit.ly/bodyplanstarter

It's essential that you select foods that you really enjoy or else you won't want to stick to this way of eating for too long.

In my first three months, I did prefer to eat very simply. This was for several reasons; mainly that I didn't want to overcomplicate my routine, and I wanted to make sure that I got the process right, but I still made sure to not sacrifice flavour or enjoyment by using flavourings and condiments that enabled me to always find the food palatable.

As I've become more confident with this *Body Plan*, I've learnt that I don't need to adhere to the body builder's stereotypical staple foods of cans of tuna, protein shakes, chicken, broccoli and rice, but if you like those then go your hardest.

Protein (animal-based)

- bacon
- eggs/egg whites
- non-fat Greek yoghurt
- low-fat/ non-fat milk ricotta cheese
- cottage cheese
- protein powder (dairy based)
- chicken
- turkey
- pork
- beef
- lamb
- white fish/shrimp
- salmon (also considered a fat source)

Protein (plant-based)

- tofu
- tempeh
- almond milk
- hummus (also considered a fat source)
- nuts/seeds or butter (also considered a fat source)
- chickpeas
- lentils
- veggie burgers
- protein powders (vegan)
- quinoa
- chia (incomplete protein)
- hemp
- amaranth

- soy milk
- legumes (incomplete protein)

Carbohydrates

- porridge/oats
- sweet potatoes & pumpkin
- rice
- bread & wraps
- fruits
- pasta
- all vegetables: especially potatoes – more comprehensive list below
- artichoke
- aubergine (eggplant)
- asparagus
- broccoflower (a hybrid)
- broccoli
- brussel sprouts
- cabbage
- cauliflower
- celery
- cucumber
- endive
- fennel
- kohlrabi
- leafy greens: beet greens (chard), bok choy, chard (beet greens), collard greens, kale, mustard greens, spinach, lettuce and arugula
- mushrooms (actually a fungus, not a plant)
- okra
- onions: chives, garlic, leek, onion, shallot,

scallion (spring onion UK, green onion US), parsley
- bell peppers/capsicum/chilli peppers (biologically fruits): chilli pepper, jalapeño, habanero
- radicchio
- rhubarb
- root vegetables: beetroot/beet, carrot, celeriac, daikon, ginger, parsnip, rutabaga, turnip, radish, wasabi, horseradish, white radish
- sweetcorn
- squashes (biologically fruits): acorn squash, bitter melon, butternut squash, banana squash, courgette/zucchini, marrow/squash, patty pans, pumpkin, spaghetti squash
- tomato (biologically a fruit)
- tubers; jicama, Jerusalem artichoke, potato, sweet potato, taro, yam

Legumes (some are protein also – will differ based on individual source)

- alfalfa sprouts
- azuki beans (or adzuki)
- bean sprouts
- black beans
- black-eyed peas
- borlotti bean
- broad beans
- chickpeas, garbanzos, or ceci beans
- green beans
- kidney beans
- lentils
- lima beans or butterbean

- mung beans
- navy beans
- pinto beans
- runner beans
- split peas
- soybeans
- peas
- mange tout or snap peas

Fruits

- açaí
- apple
- apricot
- avocado (also considered a fat source)
- banana
- bilberry
- blackberry
- blackcurrant
- black sapote
- blueberry
- boysenberry
- currant
- cherry
- cherimoya (custard apple)
- coconut (also considered a fat source)
- cranberry
- cucumber
- date
- dragonfruit (or pitaya)
- durian
- elderberry

- fig
- goji berry
- gooseberry
- grape
- raisin
- grapefruit
- guava
- jackfruit
- kiwifruit
- kumquat
- lemon
- lime
- lychee
- mango
- mangosteen
- melon: cantaloupe, honeydew, watermelon
- mulberry
- nectarine
- olive (also considered a fat source)
- orange
- blood orange
- clementine
- mandarin
- tangerine
- papaya/pawpaw
- passionfruit
- peach
- pear
- persimmon
- plantain
- plum
- prune (dried plum)
- pineapple

- pomegranate
- pomelo
- quince
- raspberry
- rambutan (or mamin chino)
- redcurrant
- satsuma
- soursop
- starfruit
- strawberry
- tamarillo
- tamarind

Fats

- fish & fish oils
- avocado
- butter / margarine
- extra virgin olive oil and any other variety of cooking or cold-pressed oils
- oil nuts/seeds or butter
- olives (also a carbohydrate source)
- coconut (also a carbohydrate source)
- tahini
- salad dressings

Once you can identify the foods you enjoy eating, look at putting together a weekly meal plan based on those foods using the rules that we've discussed before.

Meal planning guidelines

1. Know your daily budget, and then for each meal.
2. Aim for a minimum amount of protein in each meal that is equivalent to your daily total divided by the number of meals you have.
3. Brainstorm the kinds of foods you'd like to eat or are practical for you to eat, depending on whether you're at work, what food storage or heating options you have access to etc.
4. Design your ideal menu plan for the first week, adhering as best as possible to the 70/20/10 rule of whole foods, questionable foods, and pure junk/treat type foods, knowing it may not always be perfect, but it's a good goal to shoot for.

Robyn's recommendations

I like to eat the same foods on repeat until I am sick of them and, to be honest, I rotate the same types of foods all the time. Every meal except for my dinners has been pretty consistent for the past two years, except when I go on holidays or the weekends where we tend to be more relaxed eating fewer meals, but more volume or higher calorie. I usually enjoy a 'husband made' bacon and egg sandwich or waffles every weekend.

Take into account how busy your lifestyle and schedule is and how much variety you actually require. I've purchased so many fancy diet meal plans over the years, and they often need the purchase of many ingredients that are single use and then can spoil before even getting the chance to consume them, so bear that in mind.

This is why I have no problem with eating the same meals, as long as they're tasty and satisfying, I don't really mind.

It also makes it much easier for when I prepare my chicken and vegetables in bulk. Sometimes my family don't want to eat my way so if I have already made my food at the beginning and middle of the week, then I can focus purely on making their dinners each night without feeling overwhelmed that I have to prepare two lots of meals.

I've also become more efficient at making similar meals or breaking recipes down into components, like spaghetti Bolognese that I prepare for the whole family, but I might eat mine on vegetables or zucchini pasta, and the family might enjoy it on spaghetti so that I don't have to create two different meals.

Flavourings and condiments

You can use these suggested flavour enhancers to help spice up your meals but include them when logging your food as consuming too much can really bulk out your calorie spend depending on what condiments you use.

- vinegar/balsamic vinegar
- mustard
- salsa
- low-fat mayonnaise
- ketchup/tomato sauce
- marinara sauce (tomato based not seafood)
- capers
- lemon juice
- lime juice
- cinnamon
- soy sauce
- teppanyaki sauce

- hot sauce
- nutritional yeast
- other spices
- salt and pepper

Smart swaps that you won't notice

As I mentioned earlier about swapping out the pasta for vegetables or zucchini pasta which I make in a spiraliser (vegetable slicer) this is a perfect way to reduce your calories, but increase your food volume. When you start to see and experience the calorie volume of foods, you will be so amazed and understand how easy it was for you to gain weight in the first place. I couldn't believe how high-calorie a tiny portion of pasta was, and I knew it wouldn't fill me up as an entire meal.

Not only can you swap out the high-calorie ingredient entirely, but you can also play with ratios like half and half, or even one third and two thirds. I still enjoy the taste and texture of real spaghetti, so sometimes I will add a little to my zucchini noodles, so I don't feel I am missing out. Adding the zucchini creates more density to my meal, so I really feel full and satisfied without the guilt that sometimes follows an indulgence.

Use broth or water instead of oil for sautéing or cooking.

Spray oil or lightly brush a pan rather than using dollops of oil. I highly recommend acquiring a refillable pump that you can fill with your cooking oil of choice.

Low-fat or low sugar/no sugar creamer for your coffee until you are able to eliminate your milk completely. Yes, dairy milk isn't that high when you make the coffee yourself, but when you have a latte or cappuccino consisting of mostly high-fat dairy, or you use higher fat creamers like coconut milk, throughout a day these calories add up. I enjoy black coffee these days; I usually have two to three coffees a day, and sometimes I will enjoy a

Coffee-mate low sugar flavoured creamer. This is most definitely considered to be in my 10 per cent junk food as it's apparently not a high-quality food to indulge in all day, for optimum health.

A word about diet foods

As I've already outlined, with my suggested template of eating 70 per cent whole foods, 20 per cent questionable foods and 10 per cent junk foods, I know you're curious about diet foods.

Diet foods, in my belief, are foods that are man-made and manipulated, mostly to reduce fat or sugar and often use some form of artificial sweeteners to keep the calories lower than if real sugar was used. Diet foods consist of diet sodas, diet jelly (jello), coffee creamers, low-fat, no-fat or sugar-free products and artificial sweeteners.

Overall, my intuition tells me, these types of foods aren't the most significant ways to get your sources of energy.

In a perfect world, we'd all eat grass-fed meats, poultry and wild fish, plenty of fruits and vegetables that we'd grow ourselves with no pesticides, bake our own bread and consume little to no processed foods.

However, temptation is all around us these days, and it's just not practical to aim for perfection in the society that we've been brought up in.

When it comes to diet products, I exercise common sense and class them in the junk section of my daily diet. Sure, I enjoy diet drinks now and then. I sometimes use no-calorie maple syrup in my flex bowls (yoghurt, protein powder, rice crackers and syrup) and on the weekend, on my waffles. I occasionally splurge on fat-free or sugar-free flavoured creamer in my coffee when I'm tired of drinking it black. If I have a sweet craving, depending on my calorie budget for the day, I may use an artificial sweetener in my hot beverage, and I may seek out other diet products periodically. But I don't construct my whole diet out of them.

As far as my research has taken me, there doesn't appear to be enough long-standing research to suggest that some if not all of these diet products are harmful in small doses, however, I don't particularly want to experiment on myself to find out. I err on the side of caution and keep my diet products to a minimum, but don't rule them out altogether.

Robyn's recommendations

If you're currently having a love affair with diet products and a large portion of your diet consists of them, here are some of my suggestions for reducing them:

- focus on cutting them down rather than eliminating them all together, especially at first. You can aim to remove them all together if you wish in the long run, however, take it a step at a time. For example, slowly wean yourself off the artificial sweetener in your coffee. In time you might find you start to enjoy it less sweet. I used to drink tea with two sugars, now I can't even handle any sweetener, real or artificial, as I've now acquired the taste for it without, or
- try crowding out your diet products with higher quality alternatives. For example, instead of several diet sodas throughout the day, experiment with flavouring soda water with fresh lemon juice or food grade essential oils.

Cheat or treat?

If you've been on a diet before, chances are you've heard of the term cheat meal, or cheat day?

You might also be wondering how and where in your meal plan are you to place your cheat meal or day?

Well, first of all, I want to challenge you to think a little differently. The term cheat denotes that you are scamming yourself or your current eating habits and I just don't think that's a healthy mindset to breed, for a long-term lifestyle shift.

You should enjoy fun foods occasionally as part of your ongoing *Body Plan,* and including them will spell the difference between staying in for the long-haul or not. As I've mentioned previously, it's not recommended that you rely on willpower to guide you through this shift, because it is a finite resource and once depleted, you're rampant. It's also not advisable to restrict yourself from your favourite foods, because the longer you do that, the more chance of you overindulging in them.

Also, in my experience when you deprive yourself all week or month for that elusive *cheat meal*, you're likely to have little to no self-control. Sometimes just the very fact you're calling a cheat meal is harmful and can tend to demonise the food when all it is, is energy.

Making foods forbidden can create an unhealthy relationship with food which is likely to be where your problem with your weight began in the first place.

Robyn's recommendations

Don't put your favourite indulgent, fun foods on a pedestal by building up to enjoying them infrequently. We don't want to encourage a restrictive mindset surrounding food so that you start to define foods as either good or bad.

Do allocate room in your daily or weekly calorie budget to enjoy (not cheat on) some of your favourite foods. For example, I know leading up to my period's arrival I am most definitely going looking for the dark chocolate stash in the back of the freezer, and carbs are often all I feel like, but that's ok, because I allow for it and never do I allow any guilt or shame at all. Why feel shame when you can be immersing yourself in the delicious taste of your favourite food.

Trigger foods

Trigger foods are specific foods that you over-eat to the point of no control and surprisingly are not set off by cravings, emotions or your environment.

It is merely them being present that makes them hard to resist.

They are always extremely palatable, most likely highly processed, or contain the delicious combination of just the right amount of sugar, fat and/or salt.

Currently, my trigger foods are the buttercream icing I make for school bake sales or friend's birthdays or crunchy roast potatoes. Even wood-fired pizza. Yum. I can eat all these foods until I am completely stuffed. And then some.

Trigger foods are a food that once you take one little bite of, there is no hope in hell that you will be able to stop yourself.

There are two ways I'd suggest you can attack your own trigger foods.

1. **100 per cent abstinence**: works initially but you don't want to develop an unhealthy fear of it permanently because you are only adding to your guilt and reaffirming them as "unhealthy", or
2. **re-introducing the trigger food slowly** into your diet

but with another food. For example, my pizza is usually accompanied by a huge salad or plate of broccoli, so I can fill up on it first.

According to Alison Kerr, *The Binge Code: 7 Unconventional Keys to End Binge Eating and Lose Excess Weight,* "*Regular consumption of forbidden foods will prevent you from bingeing on them. You'll no longer feel so deprived and miserable. You'll start to find that prohibited foods lose their sparkle.*"

Being aware of what kinds of foods you lack control over will assist you with designing a satisfying but also sustainable meal plan, that won't set you off track, and will enable you to continue it for the long-term.

Meal preparation – easy option

Jeff Cavaliere of *ATHLEAN-X™* (one of my husband's favourite guys on *YouTube* for body conditioning and inspiration from his perspective) says when it comes to eating, we all have three options. We can either eat *good, fast or cheap.*

He says, we can never have all three, but we can shoot for two of these options.

If you chose *fast* and *good* (quality) then you may have to sacrifice a few more dollars, by perhaps buying ready-made as Jeff demonstrates in this *YouTube* clip; http://bit.ly/jeff-cav-goodfastcheap

In the video, after just fathering twins and lacking time to meal prep, he illustrates how he still maintained his health goals by ordering grilled chicken and sweet potatoes in bulk from the catering section of his local *Whole Foods* store.

You may not have this exact same option where you live, but I'm sure you have something similar, just ask at your favourite supermarket or restaurant.

If good and fast are practical options for you, you can also consider a pre-made home delivery meal service which seems to be very popular these days. They take the guesswork out of the meal prep for you but just be very mindful of the quality of the food and the menus they have as they can vary immensely from company to company. Also, don't rely on the company to dictate your calorie targets to you.

One client showed me the meals and snacks she received on her meal delivery service which consisted of mostly processed and baked goods. Despite being within her calorie targets, due to the lower quality of foods, they were lower volume and just didn't satisfy her hunger.

Another friend, same build to me, selected a similar service which allocated her 1200 calories and her husband (with a similar build to my husband) on 1400 calories and it blew my brain. First of all, I would be starving on so few calories to the point that 1200 is below my BMR. It would not result in any long-term weight loss because it wouldn't be a sustainable long-term and it's unlikely I'd adhere to eating so few calories all week long, without the risk of over-eating.

And I was right. My friend informed me she was supplementing with her own snacks in the afternoon, and both she and her husband were blowing out with takeaway and drinking on the weekends.

Imagine if you could still enjoy your treats, alcohol and occasional take away all within your daily calorie budget and still achieve your goals. You can, and you will.

When you know the calorie range you should be eating, you can have a greater awareness as to how to lose weight safely and pleasantly.

If cost is a problem for you, and you need to go down the road of *cheap* and *good*, it won't be *fast*, so you'll need to think about where to buy your food in bulk and prepare it yourself.

For example, we eat way more chicken than ever before, so now I've become clever and have sourced chicken breasts that are bulk and frozen that are way more cost effective than buying fresh and in single or smaller portions.

And for the purposes of this conversation, say you were to choose *fast* and *cheap*, then it's unlikely you'll be able to select good quality foods that are within your calorie budget unless you've allowed for it. Think fast food, like *McDonalds* or *KFC*. These are *fast* and *cheap* but hardly going to let you hit your goals if eaten regularly.

Food volume and managing hunger

Ahhh, this is the part where I am going to tell you that you can eat as much food as you want! As long as you are strategic and outline your meal plan prudently ahead of time.

One of the biggest challenges for me in the past on a diet has been handling the intense hunger, and it's most often where I've failed to commit to the said program. Most other dieters struggle with this too and expect it's all part of the dieting process.

Intense hunger doesn't need to be battled during your body transformation. Of course, there may be times when you might feel slight hunger pangs, but before acting impulsively you can ask yourself several questions:

1. Are you hungry for food? Or hungry to fill an emotional need. Comfort? Boredom? Celebration?
2. Can you cut yourself a deal? Example: you can have that piece of chocolate cake once you've eaten the massive bowl of chicken salad. Or how about sharing a portion with your kids, partner or friend?
3. Can you distract yourself with a non-food activity? Go for a walk, read a book, have a bath, play with

your kids, do some push-ups/burpees/air
squats/jumping jacks?

4. Can you come up with a low-calorie alternative to
what you're hungry for?

As already mentioned, ensuring your foods are full of fibre
which is mostly whole-grains, fruits and vegetables will give you
feelings of fullness and satisfaction.

Your goal, especially while in a *calorie deficit*, is to construct a
personalised meal plan that is full of as much volume as possible, keeping in mind your personal tastes, with as low calories as
possibly maintainable. Balancing your need for nutrients, fibre
and joy! Ha ha – see what I mean about it being as much an art
as it is a science.

Eating with such freedom and choice will take time to
finesse, but as your confidence grows, and your jeans get looser,
you'll wonder how you ever tried losing weight any other way.

Manage your intake – using the food scale

It's now a habit for both my husband and me to have our own
food scale sitting with us on the table for our meals. We had to
buy our own so that we didn't have to wait for the other to finish
weighing their food while our dinner goes cold.

Using a scale is preferable to eye-balling the quantities of
food you are consuming, at least initially, because the eye can lie
and usually if you're coming from a past of over-eating, you may
not have any idea how much you should be eating.

Also using a food scale is preferable to using volume
measurements like cups, teaspoons, tablespoons etc. because a
heaped tablespoon of peanut butter is going to yield a different
calorie result to a level tablespoon and it's tough to ensure this is
as accurate as possible unless you weigh it.

It may seem a bit pedantic, but as I've shared with you previously regarding fat yielding a higher calorie content per volume (nine calories per gram) compared to protein and carbs (four calories per gram), that extra heap of nut butter can be the difference between adherence to your calorie budget or blowing over. And over a few meals per day it can really add up.

It's not to say that you shouldn't use volume measurements (cups, teaspoons, tablespoons etc.) as sometimes you have no choice due to the food labels or the way the data is recorded in your calorie tracker app, but wherever possible, please weigh your food.

How to make it part of your day

As I've talked about previously, you'll need to work out what works best for you when it comes to remaining consistent with your own planning, logging and tracking. But one thing that has stood out with my personal experience and the clients I've worked with is those that plan ahead of time tend to have the most success.

When you take away the need of always having to think ahead to your next meal, then the stress is removed and the risk of you not adhering to your budget is reduced or eliminated.

Try to make planning ahead for the following day as routine as brushing your teeth. This is something (I hope) you do on a regular basis, without too much resistance.

The same can be done with planning the next day's meals. From a bigger picture, with regards to meal planning, I mostly bulk cook and prepare those foods that can last a few days to a week in my fridge. Things like grilled marinated chicken breast for lunches and dinners, Mexican chicken and vegetables, stir-fries, steamed vegetables, hard boiled eggs for snacks and sandwiches, and other multi-serving one pot meals that either my husband and I share or are just for me.

When it comes to planning out the following day's meals, I usually will set aside ten to thirty minutes before going to sleep to sketch out my foods for the next day. Because I tend to eat the same foods for breakfast right up to dinner, it's usually not that difficult, but as my calorie budget may change from week-to-week, it's just a matter of tweaking the volume of foods and ensuring I get adequate protein.

I pre-plan my following day's foods in my calorie tracker app, but you can even write them on a piece of paper and place that on your fridge. If you need to pack food to go, do it the night before, so it's ready for you without much thought the following day.

Logging when eating out

People who have the most success with this kind of transformation make their own meals more often than not, but I understand it's not practical to have to always eat at home, and it's a bit boring too.

Ideally, for the most part, if you can make your own meals as much as possible, and only consider eating out occasionally, if you genuinely want to change your behaviours with food and your body, then doing this will fast track your success.

However, I've had clients who have cafeteria meals at work provided to them as part of their salary package, and others that socialise heavily as part of their job. It's not as easy to adhere to their plan, but it can be managed.

The more you get into the habit of logging, weighing and tracking at home, the more confident you'll become with eyeballing the weight and calorie values of different foods.

Often, I frequent the same restaurants to eat and order the

same or similar meals, as I already have them in my personal database from the first time I went there, which makes logging so much easier.

Don't be afraid to ask your server or chef for the weight of the foods, for example: "what size steak was that?", "how much chicken did you put in the vegetable burrito bowl?" or "do you know the weight of the fish?"

Most chefs are familiar with the volume of the foods they are serving, as they are often responsible for the costing of food in the kitchen, so it's not a strange thing to ask.

I've been tempted to take a little scale with me when my calories have been quite tight but haven't got the confidence to do so just yet. I think, for now, just estimating is ok.

You can also use the guidelines I share in the *Visual Guide for Portion Control* further in this chapter.

I've been known to bring back popcorn containers from the movies, to measure the weight of my own, freshly made popcorn at home, so in future, I can estimate the popcorn calorie value for the next time I go to the movies. I can't go past popcorn and a frozen yoghurt at the movies.

I've even brought home take away French fries from the Rugby Club and weighed them too. This highlighted to me how I had been previously underestimating them.

When eating out, be mindful of extra oils, sauces and high-calorie additions to your meals. Don't be afraid to do a Meg Ryan as made famous in the 1989 movie, *When Harry Met Sally* and modify your meal as much as the restaurant will allow. Things like:

- swap French fries for a baked potato,
- ask for butter and sour cream on the side, so you can measure out your own servings or omit altogether,
- fill yourself up on vegetables or order extra,

- order two smaller starter meals or share a large meal,
- order double veggies instead of French fries,
- go for grilled or baked over fried,
- try to select meals where you can precisely determine visually what the components are of each ingredient: for example grilled protein with side salad/vegetables and a starchy non-fried carb like rice or baked potato, rather than risotto or pasta dish which is all cooked together,
- use mindful eating: eat slowly and observe when you're close to feeling full but not overly, so you don't overdo it,
- don't go crazy on the bread basket or starters, unless they're quality or worth it,
- be wary of drinking your calories as your drinks add up very quickly. Why not drink lemon infused sparkling or still water, or a diet soda? I'll talk more about how to handle alcohol further in this chapter, and
- remember that fat is nine calories per gram as opposed to protein and carbs that are four calories per gram, so prioritise your protein and carbs as it's easier to over-consume fat, especially when eating out.

If eating out doesn't occur every night of the week, you can plan ahead to allow more calories on that day or night by reducing your calorie intake by fifty calories each day to give you an extra 300 calories to enjoy in your favourite restaurant. The most critical total is that of your weekly calorie intake, not so much your daily calorie total. We just measure it daily as it's easier to manage. I'll show you how to do this in more detail in *Chapter 6: Sustain Your Progress.*

Some restaurants will have their menus online, or you can call up ahead of time to request a special meal. If those with allergies can do it, so too can you.

Don't feel the need to eat everything on your plate and if necessary, take a doggy bag home with half your meal, and it can be your lunch or dinner for the next day, primarily if it was a high-quality meal choice.

When it all comes down to it, just do the best you can, and enjoy yourself.

How to log and track multiple serve recipes

Often, I will prepare a meal for my whole family that consists of several ingredients which makes the measuring and logging of calories a little more challenging, but not impossible. It just takes a little practice and forethought.

When I am not cooking dishes where my husband and I can weigh components separately, like marinated chicken breast, stir-fried broccoli, steamed rice and sweet potato which are all cooked and served independently to make weighing each item easier, then this is what I do:

Step 1: I create the recipe in my favourite calorie tracker (at the time of publishing I have been using the premium version of *Lose It* for almost two years, so I have a very full database of recipes)

For example, if I am making Scott Baptie's Peanut Chicken from his *High Protein Handbook #4: Slow Cooker Special*

Recipe book available here http://bit.ly/scottbaptie

I input all the following ingredients into a recipe in *Lose It.*

- 1kg chicken breast, diced

- 1 onion, chopped
- 2 cloves garlic, crushed
- 120g peanut butter
- 1 tbsp cornflour
- 400g can of chopped tomatoes
- 1 red chilli, deseeded
- 2 tbsp lime juice
- 1 tbsp curry powder
- 2 tbsp soy sauce

Step 2: When the entire meal is complete, then I weigh the meal as a whole in a serving container (minus the weight of the container of course) as the total weight with the total sum of all the calories for the meal. I input this weight as servings as *Lose It* doesn't allow the option to input as grams.

Example: 750g total size of the meal, I input this as 750 servings.

Then every time I serve up a portion, I weigh the serving size, enter the value of the serving in *Lose It* (remembering it's servings in place of grams) and then determine the calories based on my serving size.

You'll need your maths brain switched on for this, and art and English were my favourite subjects, not maths, but if I can do this, then I'm confident you can too. It just takes a bit of practice and common sense, but you'll get there.

This method works well for one pot meals and slow cooker recipes that have all the ingredients placed in the one final dish.

After months of eating different variations of the same old chicken, rice or potatoes and broccoli, I finally discovered more adventurous recipes that were higher protein, super tasty and still fit within my calorie budget. My tastebuds were happier with the refreshing additions to my cooking repertoire.

If you use *My Fitness Pal*, you may find some full recipes are already input, especially those of my favourite high protein recipe creator as mentioned earlier, Scott Baptie. His online recipe eBooks contain a barcode that can be scanned directly into the *My Fitness Pal* app, if you print them, however, I prefer to input my own meals because the volume/weight of ingredients, especially whole foods (foods in their most natural and whole state) like carrots and zucchini, can change from season to season.

But please don't get hung up too much on the calorie count of non-starchy vegetables, because they really are such a low-calorie anyway, just do your best.

Unit vs quantity

I mostly weigh my vegetables, rather than selecting the quantity of said vegetable. For example, 500g of zucchini instead of one whole zucchini. It won't radically shift your total daily calorie spend unless you plan to eat a kilogram of carrots in one hit, so I wouldn't get too stressed about making sure you've input it correctly, but I just wanted to share with you my preference.

Where you will notice a difference in volume versus weight is with starchy carbohydrates or fats. For example, a small banana might only weigh 80g (72 calories) whereas a large one might be 136g (121 calories). Avocado can also trip you up depending on the size of the avocado. Half a small avocado compared to half a large one can be the difference between reaching your calorie targets or overshooting them. Remember, fat sources are nine calories per gram so can really add up.

If you're going to eat something like a chicken noodle stir-fry where all ingredients generally are cooked together, you can be a little inventive and prepare and serve the protein portion (chicken) separate to the vegetables and then the noodles (carbs) separately. This can allow everyone to serve their own meal choice which will help with personalised requirements and logging.

This is a great way my husband and I have found we can enjoy the same meal with different calorie and macronutrient requirements. He always has more calories and carbs to play with. Lucky him.

It might seem more work to initially cook this way, but this is where cooking in bulk and keeping leftovers in the fridge for next meals can save time in the long run.

Mindful eating – if you can't or won't log your food

If logging and tracking seem alien to you and it's not something you think you can sustain over a long period, then there are some other ways which can be useful. But don't forget, you won't need to track and measure forever; it's a matter of retraining yourself at first, and it's a short-term solution. But if logging your food is a concept you struggle with, there is another way. It may not be as precise and may make it harder to troubleshoot when you are not achieving results, but depending on where you are at now, it's likely to be an improvement overall.

However, personally, I prefer to have as much information as possible. I'm a bit of a data freak, can't you tell?

The purpose of logging and tracking your food intake is to help you develop your self-awareness over your current and then improved way of eating to enable you to construct balanced eating of protein, carbs and fats that are aligned with your goals. Lacking this self-awareness is likely why you've gained weight.

You've also most probably lost the ability to intuitively eat, for example knowing when to stop eating or when you're satisfied.

This has probably occurred over time due to social conditioning, peer pressure, upbringing, emotional and mental health, and stress.

Eating intuitively is tough if we've lost our connection to self, so logging and tracking can help you to reset and get a renewed understanding, as I discussed in the *Myth Busting* section in *Part I* of this book. Depending on where you are right now, just making some simple improvements will yield positive results.

Things you can focus on instead are:

- eating more consistently which basically means the same sizes and types of food as much as possible,
- eating a protein portion at every meal (snacks are also considered meals),
- only eating when you start to feel hungry even feel really hungry, also waiting to feel really hungry and just eat to feeling slightly full nothing more,
- reducing your alcohol intake,
- reducing or eliminate your eating out,
- being mindful of the oil/fat that you cook with (this can be a game changer),
- getting more sleep, and
- drinking more water.

Visual guide for portion control

- **Protein (every meal):** Women 1 palm, Men 1-2 palms
- **Starchy carbs like oats, rice, potatoes, beans, legumes, corn, pasta (1- 3 times a day)** 1-2 fists
- **Fruit and vegetable carbs (every meal when not eating starchy carbs):** Women 1 fist, Men 1-2 fists
- **Fat (most meals):** Women 1 thumb, Men 1-2 thumbs

VISUAL GUIDE FOR PORTION CONTROL

FIST

PALM

THUMB

MEN — **WOMEN**

1-2 PALMS

PROTEIN
EVERY MEAL

1 PALM

1-2 FISTS
3 TIMES A DAY

STARCHY CARBS
(OATS, RICE, POTATOES, BEANS,
LEGUMES, CORN, PASTA)

1-2 FISTS
3 TIMES A DAY

1-2 FISTS

FRUITS & VEGETABLES
EVERY MEAL WHEN NOT
EATING STARCHY CARBS

1 FIST

1-2 THUMBS

FAT

1 THUMB

Alcohol

Alcohol is sometimes referred to as the fourth macronutrient. I'm not sure why because it's not necessary for a balanced diet.

However, it might be necessary for moderation to one's lifestyle, depending on your background, culture or beliefs.

Whether you use it for social lubrication or as a way to unwind after a stressful week, it can hinder your weight loss progress if not managed correctly.

Unlike the other three macronutrients, alcohol supplies calories but absolutely no nutrition.

It's the first fuel your body will turn to, to burn off, meaning any other fuel source (carbs, protein and fats) will be stored until all the alcohol is burnt off, which will stall fat loss.

Alcohol is seven calories per gram compared to protein and carbs at four calories per gram plus it's less satisfying to your appetite, so it's much easier to over-consume, without feeling full.

It isn't necessary to abstain from alcohol completely to achieve your weight loss goals, but bear in mind the lack of nutritional benefits of consuming it and how it will eat up your calorie budget a lot faster than eating nutrient dense food will.

Not to mention the calorific foods you crave following a night on the booze. The obligatory fry up and home delivery carb and fat fest post drinking session, unless you have iron clad will. Unfortunately, I don't.

Alcohol of course also lowers inhibitions, and the relaxed feeling will make your subsequent choices less in line with your goals, so boozing regularly is likely to set your goals back.

To booze or not booze, that is the question.

This is really a very personal decision when it comes to

weight loss, and you'll need to consider what you can see your-self doing over the long haul or even short-term too.

Here's my experience.

When we first moved to Bahrain from Saudi Arabia, it was such a novelty that my husband and I could finally enjoy a few drinks after eight years of living in alcohol-free Saudi.

For the first few months, even during the week, I'd greet my husband at the door with a kiss and a can of ice-cold beer while enjoying my own mid-week cocktail of choice, usually a piña colada. Often, we'd enjoy wine with our dinner, continuing to finish the bottle while mindlessly watching late night television. We even made up for those eight lost years living in a country devoid of bars and nightclubs, by painting the town red and going out for dinners more often than we ever had before. Mostly paired with alcohol.

When I first embarked on my Body Plan, I didn't give up alcohol entirely. But I didn't want to feel unnecessary hunger and in turn waste my daily calorie budget on drinking that wouldn't satisfy my hunger. So, I rationed my drink passes to one night a week, by prioritising my social events.

I saved myself for the end of the week ritual, heading to the local Rugby club, where my girlfriends and I would share a bottle of wine, and the kids would play soccer.

I would also savour my drink by diluting it with soda. I could get more drink for my budget, while still enjoying its social lubrication.

I also reframed by focusing on my friends' company and the conversation more than the buzz.

Due to my food logging, I was also able to plan an allowance for my burger too, without any feelings of guilt, all while achieving my body goals.

After a couple of weeks of very loose logging and tracking over Christmas festivities (wine!) and hosting visiting family, I desired an alcohol break for January, not for weight control, but honestly for the relief from hangovers.

The definition of insanity is doing the same thing over and expecting different results. I truly wanted every day to feel at my best. This getting older thing has meant that my hangovers, no matter how little booze I consume, last sometimes half a week. And that fuzzy head. Not my favourite kind of feeling.

So, after a dry January, it continued, into February, March, even April with pretty much no drinking without much thought.

I had half a bottle of wine on Valentine's Day and no more than one or two drinks now and then.

I never say never, because that's just asking to be tested.

In short, at this stage, I'd rather spend my calorie budget on yummy food and not the short-lived buzz.

Robyn's recommendations

Depending on your current average alcohol consumption, consider reducing it to one night per week or reduce the volume you drink or keep it to the weekends only.

You may even wish to modify the drink you favour:

The lowest calorie options are:

- wine, which is even lower when you dilute with low-calorie lemonade or soda to reduce alcohol content,
- low-calorie beers which are similar to a glass of wine, and
- white spirits like vodka or gin, but once you mix with sodas or juice, they become higher calorie. Soda or low-calorie sodas are your best mixer option.

If you know ahead of time that you have a special occasion

coming up that involves drinking, consider one or more of the following:

- save calories over the week that you can add to your special event, e.g. if your daily calorie budget is 1700 calories you can reduce your calories by 100-150 per day to add to your event day. Remember what counts is what your total week calorie expenditure is,
- aim to keep your calories lower for the rest of the day of the event or the following day, or both,
- consume mostly protein that day, and save your carbohydrate and fat calories for your alcohol intake instead,
- alternate water or low-calorie sodas with your drinks,
- fast all day until the event or have a little protein meal right before so you don't get drunk on an empty stomach,
- be responsible – don't overdo it! and,
- enjoy yourself. If you do overdo it, congratulations you are human. Learn from it and move on. Now and then isn't going to halt your progress but a trend of going crazy on the booze might need modification.

What's more important: calories or macros?

They both serve their purpose but if you find by the end of the day that you have already reached your calorie budget total, but you have not met your daily protein target, don't attempt to eat more protein. This will send your calories into surplus which is not conducive to weight loss.

The law of weight loss is that you need to eat less energy than you are burning off. The second most important thing is to consume adequate protein.

If you find you are consistently undershooting your protein, then you need to revisit your eating behaviours and your meal planning. But if it's occasional, no problem, just aspire to do better tomorrow.

As I've mentioned with the *Twinkie diet*, Mark Haub still lost weight and was not consuming much protein at all, just plenty of fat and carbohydrates.

Did he look toned (retain muscle)? Who knows, but ideally the protein is going to help you look and feel better and help your body to perform better too as well as keep you feeling fuller for longer.

Order of importance

Calories > Macros > Training = weight loss

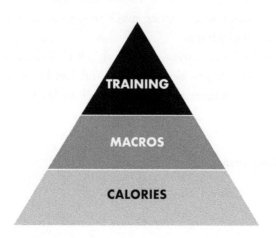

1. Forecast your daily/weekly unique energy (calorie) needs based on your goal (weight loss): **CALORIE BUDGET**
2. Establish your preference for when you prefer to eat (e.g. 5 times a day vs three larger meals a day etc.): **EATING FREQUENCY**
3. Establish your preference for what to eat of your personal food favourites and eating habits (e.g. high-fat vs high carb, etc.): **EATING PREFERENCE**

4. Determine and adhere to macronutrient targets:
   MACRONUTRIENTS BALANCE

Meal prep and planning, especially with a family that won't be eating the same way

As I've alluded to earlier, I don't always eat the exact same meals as my children, or even my husband at times.

Initially, I thought this would be a problem, as naturally most of us are time poor and having to make separate meals is just another task we don't need on our never-ending to-do list.

However, you can be smart about this and make it work for everyone.

Meal planning for my entire family was something I resisted for years, and only just recently have I even adopted the practice of making the kid's lunchboxes the evening before. Can you imagine how much that has helped with the crazy morning chaos that I thought was just the standard when raising small humans that need to get out the door five days a week to get to school on time (and with shoes on!). This has been a game changer.

But back to the meals. Most days I plan our meals in similar or different versions using the same components. As I'm not a nutritionist, I can't speak from the needs of all kids, but I follow their lead. Their energy demands more carbs than I. So, for example, if I make a Bolognese sauce (usually with plenty of hidden vegetables), then I will serve it over pasta for them, and often with garlic bread. Depending on my calorie allowance I will reduce my intake or not have any at all. Also, my children, like their father, inhale rice with their main meals, and I tend to bulk my meals out more with lower calorie but voluminous vegetables.

Every weekend, I loosely plan and prepare as much as

possible of the following weekday meals and write them down in a planner. We usually enjoy leftovers of these meals for lunches, and then we tend to go out to eat for the other meals or eat very simple thrown together meals.

The best advice I can give here is to prepare as much of your own food ahead of time as possible so that your meals are taken care of, so you'll have no excuse not to stay on track. If your family love those foods too, by all means, share it (and thank your lucky stars!) but if not then you free yourself up each day to make fresh meals for your family. Or else spend half a day on the weekend, or whenever possible, bulk prepping most meals for everyone to eliminate decision fatigue and only dirty your kitchen once or twice.

Robyn's recommendations

Allocate one or two half days throughout the week where you can dedicate your time to meal planning and bulk prepping components of your meals for the week ahead. I like Sunday mornings and Wednesdays. Prepare your lean proteins, wash and cut your vegetables, precook as much as you can ahead of time, so you cut down on the meal prep 'in the moment'.

Recipes and sample meal plan

I was at first, hesitant to share my recipes with you, because the nature of this way of eating and living, doesn't restrict you from eating anything you desire.

However, I'm sure I'd be remiss if I didn't share the foods that are on high rotation in our household, for their ease to prepare, ability to be bulk prepped and eaten as well as being delicious in taste!

For your convenience, I created a free ebook of my favourite recipes and sample meal planner which you can download here http://bit.ly/bodyplanrecipes

The nutritional stats supplied are approximate only, so make sure you input your own recipes as you make them to ensure accuracy with logging and tracking your intake.

Please bear in mind this is just a starting point for you to get your own juices flowing and to learn how to construct your own ideal meal plan that takes into account your personal tastes and preferences.

CHAPTER 6: SUSTAINING YOUR PROGRESS

*S*o many diets and fitness regimes end up failing because there's no sustainable plan for making the new habits you've created during the 'new diet' phase, actually stick. I've been there, done that, as have many of you I'm sure! So how to make these changes long-term? Well, I have quite a few strategies that I've developed that have worked for my clients and me. See what you think.

Which of them can you incorporate into your new lifestyle?

- checking in weekly,
- dealing with a plateau,
- handling your social life,
- being wise with your holidays,
- handling your 'off-season',
- rebounding after making poor choices,
- managing your daily calorie budget versus your weekly budget,
- troubleshooting your scale weight,
- the importance of maintaining consistency,
- troubleshooting your food logs, and

- planning ahead for special events.

Weekly check-in

Every week, on the same day, you will continue the process of taking your weight, body fat percentage (optional), measurements and ideally photos. This should be at a consistent time and day that you can maintain every week and have adequate time to analyse the results.

If you're maxed out during the week, but you can devote thirty minutes or more on the weekend to look over your data and determine next week's goal, then opt for a weekend. If Monday is best for you because your kids are in school and you can manage your time better, then do it then.

Mornings are preferable but work out what works best for you. The most important thing is that you're consistent with your time of day and that you do this part.

Robyn's recommendations

Every week;

- measure your weight and body fat percentage,
- take your body measurements, and
- take your progress photos.

Depending on your weekly results or your calorie budget adherence, you'll need to have a play around with your own findings based on the following (loose) guidelines.

This is where having your own coach can really help to fine-tune and troubleshoot your own personal goals and challenges.

Consider the following;

- If you lost over 500g/1 lb and didn't feel overly starving and your mood was great, you didn't feel super deprived or stressed, then stick to the same calorie and macro targets for the following week and again monitor how you feel,
- If you lost under 500g/1 lb and were not able to stick to your calorie and macro goals, then try one more week of working to these same targets (no change). If there is a pattern of your targets still being too challenging to adhere to over the next one to two weeks, then perhaps your meal planning or tracking may need to be scrutinised or problem-solved. If you're not feeling satisfied and you're not losing any weight, then there is a problem, and you'll need to understand more, by auditing your current eating habits, noticing any trends, being honest with your intake, and going back to the drawing board with your meal planning, or
- If you didn't lose anything but you were compliant to your calories, and didn't feel hungry, moody, deprived or miserable consider dropping your calories by five per cent for the next week, keeping everything else the same.

It's also a good idea, to get a holistic understanding of what else is going on for you. Return to your journal and revisit the following if significant and address as needed:

- how has your week been? Has it been any different to a typical week?
- your hunger levels,
- moods,
- energy levels,

- experiencing cravings for particular types of foods,
- sleep / rest,
- menstrual cycle,
- injuries,
- fitness / strength,
- motivation,
- stress,
- did you find it difficult or easy to stick to your calorie budget? If it was easy, were you compliant? Or did you go over?
- if you went over, what was your average calorie intake?

How to deal with a plateau

Coping with a plateau isn't something I want to cover in great detail in this book because within the first three months it's unlikely you will experience any long-term plateaus unlike if you have been on a long-term transformation like I have. And honestly, aren't you already overwhelmed enough with everything I've outlined in this book?

I will go into greater detail in my following book, but just know that plateaus are normal and to be expected if you're on a long-term path to greater health and weight loss.

This means if you have quite a bit of excess weight to lose, to do it properly and sustainably, with tools and processes that will stand the test of time and that will ensure you don't rebound, then you will need to appreciate that your weight loss will not be linear. No one wants to put in all this hard work only to have to do it all again and usually with a lot more intensity.

Our bodies are highly adaptable, and once we make changes over a while, they get used to what we are doing whether that's over-eating or severely restricting our food.

Our bodies want us to remain at our comfortable place, called homeostasis or set point.

This is why when we first try dieting, we may feel slightly hungrier as our bodies aren't quite sure what to do with this change and want us to revert back to where it was comfortable and familiar.

Over time, if we need to lose a decent amount of weight, our bodies will create multiple set points along our journey.

These set points are places that our body becomes happy to remain at, and you'll find over the years you will have experienced comfort body weights that your body tended to return back to and stay in.

When you are losing weight, your body needs time to recalibrate and create a new set point, so being able to remain at a weight for some time is part of the natural process. It will enable your body to adapt to this weight so that it will become your new and improved set point.

How to deal with socialising

Socialising for most people is one of the joys of living, and if you've ever put yourself through a torturous diet regime, you may be familiar with the loneliness it can bring about. Sometimes it might just be easier to abstain from socialising altogether, you decide. Or if you do, you may feel the unnecessary pressure from well-meaning friends to join in with some drinking or eating foods that aren't aligned with your goals.

Initially, of course, I did need to make modifications to my social life; by being mindful of the invitations I said yes to and how I would tactfully decline others. But overall, I ensured I still had some fun along the way so that I wouldn't feel deprived or suffer for my ultimate goal. You gotta enjoy the ride too.

I discussed this in greater detail in the *Soul* section, the period my husband called *The Waiting Room*, but I don't believe you should quit living your life on your way to your new *body*, *mind* and *soul*.

However, you need to understand and appreciate if you desire a change you need to enforce a difference. The way you approach this will be meaningful.

Feeling deprived will wear on your willpower over time, and you'll likely end up despising the prison you've locked yourself in.

By the same token, you won't achieve your goals if you don't reduce or modify how you socialise so here are some tips that I personally used in the beginning and still use today.

- focus on the social aspect and the relationship rather than the food or drink and also the getting ready, feeling good, doing your hair and make-up nicely,
- be a food snob, as one of my clients suggests. If you're going to enjoy something fried or indulgent, make sure it's worth it. If you have one bite, and it's not perfect and delicious don't eat it,
- the same client also makes a habit of putting her glass down regularly so she's not tempted to drink unconsciously, and often she'll forget where she put it down or lose it anyway. She'll also load up her wine with lots of ice to dilute it,
- don't announce to everyone what you're doing. It's rare that people will notice that you're not drinking or eating as much as they are until your body starts to show the results, so keep it close to your chest, and don't make a big deal about it,
- if you're struggling at a party or an event, try thinking about how you can be of service rather than eating nervously – strike up a conversation with someone

who looks like they need it, go keep the kids happy and occupied, help clear the dishes or offer to hand out the canapés,

- eat beforehand, so you don't make poorer food choices out of hunger,

- offer to be the designated driver,

- ration your alcohol by dilution. I sometimes enjoy a white wine spritzer, or vodka and soda. The drunker everyone else gets the less attention is paid to your lack of drinking,

- prioritise your social events. Do you really need to go out three times this week? No judgment but just saying. Prioritise events and focus on other non-eating/drinking activities that you can do either on your own or with a friend,

- navigate social events to be an activity instead of passive eating, e.g. meet a friend for a walk, workout and chat (one of my favourites!), go get your nails done together. Brainstorm ways you can still get your little social life box ticked without the temptation,

- have a support buddy, similarly to Alcoholics Anonymous. If you have someone close to you that you trust and that understands where you're at and is in full support of your goals, then politely excuse yourself from the party or bar, and give them a text. Or call. Distract yourself, and

- if all else fails then just enjoy the event. One bad meal or occasion won't make you fat, just like one salad won't make you lean. It's all about what you do the majority of the time.

How to deal with holidays

Family vacations or holidays with friends are one of life's greatest pleasures but can often be the undoing of many a healthy diet and lifestyle intention.

Having a game plan is essential but does not need to be limiting or joyless.

I'm a world traveller and a huge advocate or immersing yourself in the country or location you are visiting and that most definitely includes sampling the food.

I could never imagine not enjoying:

- an Afghan biscuit in New Zealand,
- a Cornish pasty in England,
- a Scooby snack in Glasgow (it's not what you think!),
- a lava flow cocktail in Honolulu,
- a few beers and complimentary snacks at a Cantina in Mexico,
- delicious chicken and rice in Cuba,
- a shawarma or chicken biriyani in Saudi Arabia,
- pasta and pizza by the truckload in Rome,
- apperitivo (nibbles in the afternoon) with my drink at a bar in Milan,
- all the delicious home comfort foods of Portugal,
- the incredible and irresistible curries and Dahl and dosas of Sri Lanka,
- the pad Thai and green chicken curry of Thailand, and
- the meat pies and ice coffees from the petrol station in my homeland Australia.

But as my trainer and friend Danielle Wilkinson says when

she talks about planning for a vacation, *"Don't be a knob head,"* when it comes to going on holiday. I'll explain more below.

Robyn's recommendations

Before you go away you will need to ask yourself a few questions;

- how long are you going away for? A shorter trip can allow a little more leeway whereas a more extended holiday may require some forethought,
- who are you going away with? A family trip may be a little different to a wild cruise away with girlfriends, who are dead set on drinking the trip away,
- what is your accommodation like? Will you have access to a kitchen or will your food be supplied? Will you be eating out all the time?
- what kinds of foods do you think you'll have access to? Remember, depending on where you are going and what types of facilities you'll have available will impact this. Use *Google* to seek out supermarkets or even menus of restaurants or accommodation if possible, and
- how active will your holiday be? Will you be walking, riding, doing much activity or will it be a lying on the beach reading a book the whole time kind of vacation?

When you have a clearer understanding of your holiday and how it is going to playout, then you can work out if you're just going to be completely switched off and relaxed about what choices you make or if you wish to have a game plan.

On a recent two-week trip to Sri Lanka, I planned to do

plenty of walking, eat a decent high protein provided breakfast and then just take each day at a time, based on where we were and what foods were on offer.

On the days we spent mostly driving (up to five hours a day) I ate very little as I wasn't being active, and I didn't require much energy. On the other days in beautiful locations with irresistible Sri Lankan curries on offer, I indulged.

After my husband would return from a surf, we'd tag-team supervising the kids on the shore, so I could have an ocean swim and do some water running. Also, when I'd swim with the kids, I'd be water running too. But fitness isn't a focus for you right now. I will discuss my approach to fitness more in the following book.

Keep in mind that in one to two weeks of a holiday it is difficult to do permanent damage unless you are a 'knob head' and completely over-eating and overindulging in alcohol and calorie dense foods and drinks, with very little activity, don't eat any vegetables and eat all the fried foods.

You can still enjoy one or two delicious and indulgent meals a day with wild abandon but just don't eat to feeling overstuffed regularly. Ensure you're getting adequate protein mostly, try to be a little active even if it's just walking up and down the beach and doing water running like me in Sri Lanka. You can also skip a meal here and there if you know you're going to be going a little more overboard one or two days.

Other tips:

- drink coffee, water or diet soda to tide you over between meals,
- select one meal per day that is going to be your favourite meal for the day and plan your eating around that. Maybe you'll be going out for a buffet dinner, so eat lighter throughout the day, or perhaps

you'll be having a special breakfast or lunch, so get
moving afterwards or eat lower carb and protein for
the rest of the day,

- eat as many meals as possible in your hotel,
apartment etc. depending on your accommodation,
- have healthy snacks readily available depending on
your set up (yoghurts, low-fat cheeses, crackers, oats,
protein shakes that can be made with water in a
shaker, fresh fruit),
- aim for a serve of protein (not fried, crumbed or
battered) at every meal, one with a salad and one
with starchy carbs like rice, or baked potato but be
mindful of any extra fats,
- eggs are great breakfast options, poached or
hardboiled are best, but fried is still ok (just
remember it's hard to know how much fat they've
been cooked in, and it can really add up), and
- aim to treat yourself one meal per day, not all meals.

**It's ok to have an off-season but don't use it as an excuse to
derail you**

When I was powerlifting with my personal trainer Alastair last
year, he taught me the importance of having time off consistent
training.

As we were both heading into the summer school holidays,
and him in the off-season from his rugby, he reminded me that
athletes have training breaks during the off-season, so they can
come back stronger and not burn out.

This is excellent advice to apply to diet as well. Especially if
you've been logging and measuring for an extended period as
I had.

Evidence-Based Training, a Swedish fitness and nutrition-based company states:

"Diet breaks appear to reverse important physiological adaptations to energy (calorie) deficit, subsequently making the dieting period following a break more effective for fat loss. Performing a diet break every four to eight weeks versus every two weeks may be a useful strategy to enhance fat loss and mitigate declines in resting energy expenditure."

This was based on a study where two groups of male dieters were put on a calorie deficit diet with the first group continuing for sixteen weeks and the second group given a break for two weeks every two weeks which took their total period of dieting to thirty weeks (sixteen weeks of dieting and fourteen weeks of non-diet break).

What was found was that both groups had effectively been in diet-mode for a total of sixteen weeks, but the second group, despite taking almost twice as long in total to complete the diet due to their diet breaks every two weeks, still lost 50 per cent more mass than the first group. So not only were they in a better position than the first group, they were able to enjoy diet breaks which aren't just great for fat loss but also for the mindset.

Taking breaks along your journey is smart if you want to see long-term results, enabling you to see out your long-term vision. When you return from your break, you'll come back mentally stronger than if you had been on the plan continuously.

The secret, however, is that during your 'breaks', try your best not to go over your maintenance caloric intake. That way, you don't gain any unwanted fat during this time.

Personally, I'd think breaks after eight, ten or twelve weeks are advisable timeframes, but once again this isn't something, I believe you'd need to enforce within your first three-month cycle.

How to rebound after a big weekend or several days of poor choices

You don't have to be perfect because nobody is perfect. We all mess up on our diets. You will, however, need to learn how to rebound in the best way possible after you've had a big weekend, or emotionally eaten, or overindulged.

Plan a *High-Intensity Interval Training (HIIT)* session, or do some *intermittent fasting (IF),* or get back on track the next day. No problem. No excuses. Just have a plan. Don't let a bad day affect you; use it to fuel your fire.

Don't use your poor choices as a reason to make even more poor decisions; use it as a reason to get back to your plan.

I love the analogy that I heard recently about accidentally dropping your mobile phone. The screen appears cracked but is still in working order. Do you then go and smash it even more? No, I didn't think so.

The most important thing to remember is that to lose weight you need to be in a calorie deficit. Even though your calorie budget is given daily, you can borrow from other days within a week. So long as your weekly total is still within your budget, you can sometimes recover your poor choices.

One hundred to 300 calories over budget are usually recoverable, especially if you can manage it over a few days; however, anything over 400 may be harder to recover, so in my opinion, I would just cut your losses and begin again today. But without any guilt. I really hope you enjoyed your big weekend or treats because guilt really is a wasted emotion. Enjoy your time for what it was, then get back on track and learn from this opportunity.

Daily calorie budget vs weekly calorie budget

By now you should already know that the most important thing for you to have success with weight loss is that you need to adhere to a safe and sustainable calorie deficit. I think I've banged on enough about this already. Whichever way you decide to achieve your calorie deficit is entirely up to you.

Knowing that not every day is the same for anyone means you will face fluctuations in hunger levels, energy resources, hormones, social obligations and even stress.

Because of this, sometimes, adhering to the same calorie budget every day of the week might prove to be a challenge. So, in order for you to not go crazy, and to empower you on those days you just know you're going to overindulge, you can borrow calories from the following day. You can even bank some extra calories from previous days for a future event if necessary.

The way I've recommended you manage your calories over a day just makes it more practical to control, which is why we set a daily target rather than a weekly target. But fundamentally, all that matters is you don't exceed your weekly calorie target.

Make sense?

For example, most weekends, I find I tend to go over my allocated budget repeatedly, so over time I have naturally eaten less over the weekdays and allocated myself more calories to enjoy the weekend festivities.

By saving fifty calories over the six days during the week, I am then able to eat an extra 300 calories over the weekend, either on one whole day (a dinner out at a restaurant or a couple of alcoholic beverages) or to split it over the two days.

I don't always do this, but this is where my planning ahead of time and knowing my schedule can really support this strategy.

Of course, some days just happen that are unplanned, and that's ok too. For example, when all good intentions are mislaid (aka the unexpected pork bun and boozy night at the Rugby club), then I just plan to do better the following day by recovering excess calories if and when possible. Just remember if you've gone really crazy like 1000 to 2000 calories over, just write it off as a good time and get back to your goals the following day. You're human, don't dwell on it, but don't become a victim to it either.

Here's how to work out your weekly budget:

Daily calorie budget x 7 = weekly budget

Example: 1500 x 7 = 10,500

This can be structured like this:
Monday: 1450
Tuesday: 1450
Wednesday: 1450
Thursday: 1450
Friday: 1450
Saturday: 1800
Sunday: 1450
Weekly total = 10,500

Or

Monday: 1400
Tuesday: 1400
Wednesday: 1400
Thursday: 1500
Friday: 1900
Saturday: 1500
Sunday: 1450
Weekly total = 10,500

Or

Endless combinations as you can see...

You can also use this strategy when starting to add or increase training into your lifestyle, to give yourself more energy on training days but as discussed, this really isn't too great a focus for you just yet.

Troubleshooting scale weight

From time to time, throughout your weekly check-in process, you may be frustrated to find that your weight is reducing over the week, but when it comes to your check-in day, it may have jumped up.

Despite me previously reassuring you that the scale weight is only one third of the puzzle giving you an accurate picture, it can be really disheartening to see your progress over the week change on the one day it really seems to count in your mind.

So, here's a suggestion, but it's only really the last resort at this point because it's not something I advise for you to start doing until you really have established your first three months on *The Body Plan*.

An option is to weigh yourself every morning at the same time, same place, same conditions, and average your weekly result. Using a free smartphone app like *Happy Scale* can take the hard work out of working out your average weight manually.

If this is not practical for you, or if you feel this could breed obsessive tendencies then skip it.

Just be mindful that small (or even seemingly large) fluctuations in scale weight overnight do not necessarily mean you have gained fat overnight. It's really not possible unless you have really gone to town with your eating.

Usually, the answer is hormones, stomach contents (undigested food), temporary water retention caused by dehydration or higher carb intake which results in glycogen storage in the body or even pump in your muscles from heavy training.

Detach your emotions from the results on the scale and use it purely as a data point to help you manage yourself moving forward.

What's essential is the overall trend of your weight reducing and your body composition. Your body composition is how toned and lean you look and feel and how your clothes fit, as you may lose centimetres while still weighing the same on the scale. From day-to-day, it's less critical. Try your hardest not to freak at the sight of a fluctuation. This is normal.

In particular, I have to regularly remind my husband of this, whenever he says on a night following a couple of slices of pizza, despite remaining within his calorie balance, he has gained 'weight'. I tell him time and time again, it's impossible to gain weight overnight from a couple of pieces of pizza, it's likely water weight or glucose storage or even he might just need to do a poo, to return him back to his usual weight.

Every four weeks, if you're a fertile woman, it's likely too that your scale is going to show a heavier weight.

My awareness of my cycle has never been so sharp since doing this *Body Plan* and being vigilant with my record keeping (it only took me to forty years of age to learn this!), and now I know without even checking my smartphone cycle tracking app, that my period is on its way. Whether it's the extra carb or chocolate craving right before or the swelling of my tummy or excess weight (usually water weight) in the week leading up to it, or my lack of strength at the gym, I've learnt to factor it into the picture.

Again, the scale reading is not the full picture; it's just a tool we use to monitor our ongoing progress. If your pants are feeling more snug than usual and you're starting to appear fluffier in the mirror then yes, perhaps you're gaining weight, but it doesn't happen overnight. Just like your dream body doesn't occur overnight too.

Consistency

If you've come from a history of yo-yo dieting, then it's likely that your lifestyle hasn't demonstrated any kind of consistency.

Perhaps you've never known from day-to-day what meals you were going to eat ahead of time, preferring to wing it, or you grabbed things on the go, or perhaps you're a chronic snacker.

Perhaps every January you hit the gym with all the other January joiners, only to give up after a few weeks, never to be seen again until next year.

Perhaps your sleep schedule hasn't been intentional, either falling asleep watching *Netflix*, or collapsing at random times without any pre-bedtime rituals.

Perhaps your eating habits have reflected your mood or emotional state at any given moment.

Being able to manage and measure your success over time will become more natural and instinctual, but if you're being inconsistent in your habits, from sleep to eating, to timing, to training, overall it's going to be difficult for you to troubleshoot when things aren't going to plan.

When it comes down to it, your weight loss is just a side effect of making ongoing, positive choices and behaviours.

Real transformation can only come about from showing up every day. Of course, there will always be one-off times that will throw off best intentions, but remain flexible and learn how to steer those situations so that you're adhering to your plan more often than most.

Earlier in this chapter, I suggested some ways that you can

play around with your calorie targets so that you have some high and low days, but at the beginning of adjusting to this new and improved lifestyle, I'd recommend you try to adhere to mostly being consistent throughout your week so that your opportunities for error are reduced.

Robyn's recommendations

Ways to be consistent can be:

- select your daily eating schedule preference and adhere to it. For example, if you prefer to eat more frequent but smaller meals throughout the day, perhaps your schedule would look similar to mine: breakfast: 630am, morning tea or post workout: 11am, lunch: 2pm and dinner 6pm,
- select your daily meal times and do it, every day,
- eat the same or similar meals each day, until you get sick of them, then swap them out for something different, and repeat the process. Not only does it help with decision fatigue and keeping compliant, but it also helps with maintaining food costs and reducing waste,
- choose one or two days a week to meal plan and prep. I really like Sundays and Wednesdays,
- have a date night or restaurant meal once a week,
- limit alcohol to one night a week, and
- be consistent in your entire approach to your self-care aka *The Body Plan*.

Troubleshooting food logging

Throughout your weight loss journey, you will find that you'll need to audit your logging and troubleshoot your results when things aren't going to plan. The purpose of logging is to self-monitor your habits and to give you a data set to scrutinise your eating habits so that you can hit your body goals. Be it that your weight loss has stalled, or you feel starving, and your calorie budget seems sufficient, but you just cannot sustain such low food intake.

It's been reported that many undercut their reported calorie intake by sometimes up to 50%. Snacking throughout the day, grabbing bites of this and that, or eating then forgetting to log your food is easily done. Many weight loss patients have struggled to lose weight, believing themselves to be in a calorie deficit, but when their accurate intake was measured in a strict lab setting, they were discovering they weren't being entirely truthful with their consumption and were either knowingly or unknowingly over-consuming thus impacting their ability to lose weight.

Snacking between meals that you disregard adds up, as does misjudging what you are eating. This is where being consistent in your eating habits, and dedicated to sticking to meal timings as often as possible, as mentioned earlier, can really help to support you and eliminate the opportunity for error.

If you're not losing weight, you'll need to return to your data and try and discover the reason.

Especially as you start losing more weight, the data you collect will become of more importance as you need to modify your food intake.

When scrutinising your data, first of all make sure it's accurate as mentioned in *Chapter 4: Understanding Flexible Dieting.*

Then ask yourself some questions:

Is my inability to be adherent to my calories happening now and then or on one-off occasions?

Is my failure to be adherent occurring frequently, and if so, is there a recurring pattern? For example, are you managing to adhere to your calorie budget throughout the week but on weekends, you're going way over? Are you compliant to your calories all month until your period is on its way?

If your inability to be adherent is happening all the time, then it's time to revisit your meal plan. Perhaps you're not feeling satisfied, and your meals are not appropriately balanced with the right amount of fat and protein to help sustain you. Or maybe you're restricting yourself from foods that you enjoy so that you end up getting to the end of the day and bingeing on them. Perhaps you haven't cleared the chaos in your life to prioritise your meal prep, or you could even be on too low calories, so that you are unable to adhere to them.

If your struggle to be compliant only happens from time to time, there are ways you can rebound with little to no impact on your goal.

I get it, life is always going to throw us curveballs, whether it's a celebration or mourning. Life, as it is, is going to test our *Body Plan* goals, and that's ok because hopefully within this book you will have the tools to know how to get back on track when this does happen.

If I've found myself at the end of the day for any number of reasons having gone over my calories but just by 100 to 300 calories, I can breathe a sigh of relief and know that I can just take those calories off the next few days, without deprivation.

What counts in the end is your weekly total as I've discussed earlier. We just break it down into daily amounts to help you manage your hunger and portion control across the week. When you start introducing training into your routine, you may even find that you wish to play around with the daily amounts, so that on or before training days, you will eat slightly more to fuel you, and on the other days you will eat less to bring your weekly total down. This isn't anything you should really worry about at this point in your journey, as I've said so many times before, your focus for the first three months is to be consistent, educated and confident with our nutrition, first and foremost.

If you've had a super indulgent unplanned event which could take you from 500 calories plus over your daily budget (yep a few times I've been over 2000 calories with a boozy, party weekend and subsequent junk food feast hangover). When that happens, it's just easy to write that day off rather than go super low on my intake for the following days which can end up disastrous and set off an under-eating and over-eating cycle.

Don't feel any guilt or shame about it, enjoy it! Don't allow that indulgence to go to waste with any unnecessary feelings of delinquency – hell no! It was fun at the time so appreciate it for the joy it brought. But don't take it as a free pass to let loose or don't make it a setback, it's not. Its life and food is life, so enjoy and rebound with the best possible mindset you can first and foremost then the rest will follow.

If you're struggling to log and track your meals, perhaps you need to return to *Part I* of this book to work on setting the foundations for your *Body Plan*. You either want results, or you'll find the reasons why you can't achieve them. It will all come back to how much you want this, and what's it going to take for you to commit to this plan.

Perhaps you're happy enough where you are, and that's perfectly fine too. Don't get me wrong, though this inner journey which has reflected on the outside, I have reached a level of inner peace and happiness too. If nothing changed, I would be happy to stay right here. Having that level of detachment has helped me to move forward, without timelines, pressure or unhealthy habits.

If you feel that logging or tracking your calories is too time-consuming, revisit where you can recover time in your day that is otherwise less productive. Reducing social media, waiting in lines, waiting to pick up kids at school, on public transport, setting it as part of your evening ritual for the day before. If you want something hard enough, you will make time for it.

Robyn's recommendations

Revisit your '*why*'. What was the reason for you to embark on this life-changing and enhancing plan? What did you visualise for yourself? Go back to the intentions you set initially in *Chapter 1: Setting Your Intentions* to get back on track.

Special events – planning ahead

When I know I have a fun dinner or evening coming up with my husband or friends, usually, I know in advance, and I can plan my weekly calorie budget around it accordingly. This works best when you know your social calendar ahead of time, but as I've also mentioned above, you can always recover from impromptu events too.

Last year I had a friend's birthday cocktail evening planned a week in advance with all the girls. A bit of mid-week fun away from the bedtime routine for all of us. It was fab.

We were going to one of our favourite bars, unlimited cocktails and ceviche (literally the best – have you tried it?!) and I knew I wouldn't be able to calorie track nor manage my intake of either, so I fasted all day in preparation.

You may have heard of *Intermittent Fasting (IF)* as a diet to lose weight, and I'm not going to go into too much detail about *IF* in this book because it's not something I used at *Phase I* in my own journey. I personally do not consider *IF* a diet on its own, but merely a tool to reduce your "eating window". I didn't begin to experiment with it until around the six-month mark in my own journey.

Of course, on this night in question, I fasted all day until right before heading out the door. I was responsible, however, and I ate some high protein food right before leaving the house and hitting the bar (I've learnt from experience in my late teens never to go out drinking on an empty stomach; I'm sure you have too) and made sure to eat some delicious ceviche before sucking back on those delightful cocktails.

A final note

Within this book, I've given you all the tools, processes and practices that I used to jump start my own body transformation which is still in operation and I imagine it will be for life, however, with time it will become (and already has to some degree) second nature.

As with anything in life, business, learning a new language, managing your finances or starting a new job, there is a learning curve. Please know you may not acquire the necessary behaviours immediately, but if you commit to you, your health and your future just a little each day and try to be better each week than you were last week, then you will be closer than you were yesterday.

There is always discomfort and resistance when embarking on something new, but if you can move through this feeling and focus on your intentions and the future you, you will be rewarded.

I have given you all I can to help kick-start you on your own journey, but ultimately it is YOU that must now do the work. I cannot do this for you. You have to believe in yourself enough and want this for you and your family to do the job. I pinkie promise it will get easier over time; don't give up before the miracle occurs.

After your first three months have been completed, you may have all you need to move forward in your own body transformation, but if you want to learn more about what I did following month three, then I look forward to sharing more with you soon.

ACKNOWLEDGEMENTS & RECOMMENDED RESOURCES

If you'd like to access this list online you can visit
http://bit.ly/bodyplanstarter

- Dr Joe Dispenza, 2012, *Breaking the Habit of Being Yourself: How to Lose Your Mind and Create a New One,* Hay House Inc.
- Traci Pedersen, Psych Central 2012, *High-Fat Diet Linked to Depression, Anxiety in Mice,* accessed on December 9, 2018, on https://psychcentral.com/news/2012/05/28/high-fat-diet-linked-to-depression-anxiety-in-mice/39295.html
- Traci Mann Ph.D, 2015, *Secrets From the Eating Lab: The Science of Weight Loss, the Myth of Willpower and Why You Should Never Diet Again,* HarperCollins Publishers.
- Susan Peirce Thompson, Ph.D, 2017, *Bright Line Eating: The Science of Living Happy, Thin & Free*, Hay House Inc.
- Henry S. Lodge M.D and Chris Crowley, 2007, *Younger Next Year for Women: Live Strong, Fit, and Sexy*

—*Until You're 80 and Beyond,* Workman Publishing Company.

- Alan Aragon, Jan 10, 2014, *10 Essential Characteristics of a Healthy Diet,* accessed December 9, 2018, by http://www.alanaragonblog.com/wp-content/uploads/2014/01/10-Essential-Characteristics-of-a-Healthy-Diet.pdf

- Jeff Cavaliere, ATHLEAN-X™, January 13, 2016 *Meal Prep Hack (30 MEALS / 30 SECONDS!),* accessed on December 9, 2018 on https://www.youtube.com/watch?v=6MR7uBRVnZg

- Gary Foster, Ph.D, Livestrong.com, *The Percentage of People Who Regain Weight After Rapid Weight Loss and the Risks of Doing So,* accessed on December 9, 2018 on https://www.livestrong.com/article/438395-the-percentage-of-people-who-regain-weight-after-rapid-weight-loss-risks/

- Walter Mishcel, 1960/1970, *The Stanford Marshmallow Experiment,* accessed on December 9, 2018 on https://en.wikipedia.org/wiki/Stanford_marshmallow_experiment

- Eugene K, Choi, October 25, 2018. *How to Attain Self Realization (Step-By-Step Guide for a Better You),* accessed on December 9, 2018 on https://www.lifehack.org/682908/how-to-attain-self-realization-a-guide-to-become-a-better-you

- Shai Danzigera, Jonathan Levavb, and Liora Avnaim-Pessoa, 2010, *Extraneous factors in judicial decisions,* accessed on December 9, 2018 on https://www.pnas.org/content/pnas/108/17/6889.full.pdf

- NHS UK, June 13, 2017, *Being overweight, not just obese, still carries serious health risks,* accessed on December

9, 2018, https://www.nhs.uk/news/obesity/being-overweight-not-just-obese-still-carries-serious-health-risks/

- Elizabeth Daniels, 2013, *How to Manifest What You Want Now*, accessed on December 9, 2018 on https://www.applythelawofattraction.com/manifest-what-you-want-now/
- Jim Fortin, October 18, 2018 *Sales Psychology with Jim Fortin Facebook post*, accessed on December 9, 2018 on https://www.facebook.com/salespsychologyacademy/photos/a.781542385207250/2309809295713877/?type=1&theater
- Elizabeth Gilbert, April 10, 2015, *Beware of Tribal Shame Facebook post*, accessed on December 9, 2018 on https://www.facebook.com/GilbertLiz/photos/a.356148997800555/806648316083952/?type=1&theater
- Maslow's Hierarchy of Needs, *Wikipedia*, accessed on December 9, 2018, on https://en.wikipedia.org/wiki/Maslow%27s_hierarchy_of_needs
- Danielle La Porte, 2014, *The Desire Map: A Guide to Creating Goals with Soul*, Sounds True Publishing.
- Julia Cameron, 2016, *The Artist's Way*, Tarcher Perigee.
- Amy B Wang, Washington Post, December 12, 2017, *Former Facebook VP says social media is destroying society with 'dopamine-driven feedback loops'*, accessed on December 9, 2018, on https://www.washingtonpost.com/news/the-switch/wp/2017/12/12/former-facebook-vp-says-social-media-is-destroying-society-with-dopamine-driven-feedback-loops/?noredirect=on&utm_term=.bc4bdbf2ca81

- Kelsey Byers, 2013, *Eat Clean and Follow Your Dreams,* CreateSpace Independent Publishing Platform
- Center for Humane Technology, *Our society is being hijacked by technology,* accessed on December 9, 2018, on http://humanetech.com/problem/
- Alexandra Franzen, August 19, 2015, *Why I don't use social media anymore,* accessed on December 9, 2018, on http://www.alexandrafranzen.com/2015/08/19/why-i-do-not-use-social-media-anymore/
- Gerald M. Weinberg, 1991, *Quality Software Management: Systems Thinking,* Dorset House.
- Four Burner Theory, November 22, 2017, *The Four Burner Theory for How to Manage Your Ambitions,* accessed on December 9, 2018, on https://heleo.com/conversation-four-burner-theory-manage-ambitions/15027/
- Zdravko Cvijeticm, Medium, *13 Things You Should Give Up if You Want to Be Successful,* accessed on December 9, 2018, on https://medium.com/@zdravko/13-things-you-need-to-give-up-if-you-want-to-be-successful-44b5b9b06a26
- Alexandra Franzen, 2017, *How to Say No (free workbook),* accessed on December 9, 2018, http://www.alexandrafranzen.com/wp-content/uploads/2017/01/how-to-say-no_free-workbook_franzen.pdf
- Carmine Gallo, Entrepreneur.com, October 14, 2011, *Steve Jobs and the Seven Rules of Success,* accessed on December 9, 2018, on https://www.entrepreneur.com/article/220515
- Dr Spencer Nadolsky, November 3, 2018, *"You don't have a slow metabolism, you eat more than you think..."*

Instagram post, accessed on on December 9, 2018, on https://www.instagram.com/p/BpuUxRAgOGC/

- CNN Health, Madison Park, November 8, 2010, *Twinkie diet helps nutrition professor lose 27 pounds,* accessed on December 9, 2018, on http://edition.cnn.com/2010/HEALTH/11/08/twinkie.diet.professor/index.html

- British Nutrition Foundation, January 2018, *Dietary fibre*, accessed on December 9, 2018, on https://www.nutrition.org.uk/healthyliving/basics/fibre.html

- Harris Benedict Equation, *Wikipedia*, accessed on December 9, 2018, on https://en.wikipedia.org/wiki/Harris%E2%80%93Benedict_equation

- Barry Schwartz, 2009, *The Paradox of Choice: Why More Is Less,* Harper Collins Publishers.

- Alison Kerr, 2017, *The Binge Code: 7 Unconventional Keys to End Binge Eating & Lose Excess Weight,* Mindfree.

- Scott Baptie, Food for Fitness, *High Protein Handbook 4,* accessed on December 9, 2018, https://www.foodforfitness.co.uk/high-protein-recipes/

- EBT : Evidence Based Training, May 10, 2018, *Diet Breaks - Instagram post*, accessed on December 9, 2018, https://www.instagram.com/p/BimlUHNgLLK/

Recommended Resources

- Digital body fat and weight scale https://amzn.to/2C8eQyH
- Tape measure https://amzn.to/2rA9giI

- Journal https://amzn.to/2EgYtBl
- Smartphone tripod https://amzn.to/2QNQhiK
- Digital kitchen scale https://amzn.to/2UBoJMA
- Calorie counter smartphone app *Lose It* http://bit.ly/bodyplanloseit or *My Fitness Pal* http://bit.ly/bodyplanMFP
- Spiraliser (vegetable slicer) https://amzn.to/2PrUnrX
- Scott Baptie, High Protein ebooks http://bit.ly/scottbaptie

FREE TOOLS

As I've mentioned throughout this book, I've put together a starter kit to complement the strategies I've shared with you and to get you started on your own journey.
You can access the starter kit here
http://bit.ly/bodyplanstarter

And don't forget to sign up to receive a free ebook of my favourite recipes and a meal plan to get you started and complement what I share in *The Body Plan*.
http://bit.ly/bodyplanrecipes

DID YOU ENJOY THIS BOOK?

If you've got a moment and you enjoyed my book, I would be very grateful if you'd spare a moment to offer a review (it can be as short as you like) on this book's Amazon page.

Honest reviews help me to bring more of what you like to you, and my work to the attention of other readers just like you.

You can jump right back to the page by visiting here

https://amzn.to/2QwUO9X

Thank you!

ROBYN LAW

Robyn Law is mostly an at-home mother and a part-time writer. Professionally she has worked in corporate finance, been a make-up artist, enjoyed an eventful decade as a domestic and international flight attendant, worked as a nanny, certified as a raw-food chef, became a professional blogger, coached women in online business and consulted on online marketing. These experiences and some extreme life adventures have brought her to writing about her latest passion, self-transformation, a process she applies to body, mind, and raising her family abroad.

You can find her online at RobynJLaw.com
or send an email to robyn@robynjlaw.com

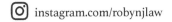 instagram.com/robynjlaw

Milton Keynes UK
Ingram Content Group UK Ltd.
UKHW011732200524
442976UK00037B/600

9 780648 477402